Tortillas, Tiswin, and T-Bones

TORTILLAS TISWIN & T-BONES

A Food History of the Southwest

Gregory McNamee

University of New Mexico Press | Albuquerque

© 2017 by Gregory McNamee
All rights reserved. Published 2017
Printed in the United States of America
22 21 20 19 18 17   1 2 3 4 5 6

Library of Congress Cataloging-in-Publication Data
Names: McNamee, Gregory, author.
Title: Tortillas, Tiswin, and T-bones : A Food History of the Southwest /
    Gregory McNamee.
Description: Albuquerque : University of New Mexico Press, 2017. |
    Includes bibliographical references and index. |
Identifiers: LCCN 2017012534 (print) | LCCN 2017014273 (ebook) | ISBN 9780826359049 (pbk. :
    alk. paper) | ISBN 9780826359056 (E-book)
Subjects: LCSH: Food—Southwestern States—History. | Food—Mexico—History. | Cooking,
    American—Southwestern style—History. | Diet—Southwestern States—History. | Diet—
    Mexico—History. | Food habits—Southwestern States—History. | Food
    habits—Mexico—History.
Classification: LCC TX360.U6 (ebook) | LCC TX360.U6 M3935 2017 (print) |
    DDC 641.300979—dc23
LC record available at https://lccn.loc.gov/2017012534

Some of this material was originally published on the *Encyclopaedia Britannica* blog,
in the *Virginia Quarterly Review*, and in various editions of *Harris' Almanac*.

Unless otherwise noted, all photographs are by Gregory McNamee.

Cover photographs: (top) courtesy of the Library of Congress;
(bottom) courtesy of Gregory McNamee
Designed by Felicia Cedillos
Composed in Minion Pro 10.25/14.25

Contents

Introduction   vii

  1. **Origins**   1

  2. **Native America**   19

  3. **Entradas**   43

  4. **La Frontera**   63

  5. **The Anglo Frontier**   81

  6. **Extending the Larder**   105

  7. **African Americans**   127

  8. **The Old World and the New**   141

  9. **Asian Americans**   157

  10. **Corporatization and Standardization**   175

  11. **Drink**   191

  12. **The Future of Southwestern Food**   209

Acknowledgments   227

References   229

Index   235

Introduction

Man cannot live by bread alone. So the Bible tells us, and the words are wise. Set a hot dog down on top of that bread, though, and the odds of survival brighten considerably. Lay on a slab of beef, a chicken breast, or—best of all, despite the dark admonitions of doctors—a pile of bacon, and instead of man's not being able to live, you have created a world in which all humankind flourishes and prevails.

One of the great insights that just about every culture on earth has had over the course of history has been that if you take some sort of bread and stuff it with some kind of filling, often but not necessarily meat, happiness will ensue. Thus pot stickers and pasties, pot pies and pocket pitas, pastrami on rye and jambon de Paris, pierogies and pupusas—and, to get away from all those plosive *p*'s, tamales, samosas, gyoza, ravioli, and good old-fashioned hamburgers.

In the American Southwest, the part of that bread with filling that produces contentment has for a very long time been played by the taco. Its overall origins lie south of the international border with Mexico, and for much of its life, the taco, when it was known at all beyond the Southwest on this side of the line, was seen as an exotic stranger. But lately, the taco has come to be a definitively all-American food—by which I mean that it has been embraced in every part of the country without qualm or question, as if it had always been part of the national cuisine. Go to Providence, Rhode Island, and you'll find some restaurant that celebrates Taco Tuesday. Travel to Point

Barrow, Alaska; or Montauk, New York; or Atlanta or Twin Falls or Dededo, and you'll find a taco stand. Moreover, because it's all-American, the taco is all-global: Our tacoshed, the geographical area that embraces our beloved foodstuff, takes in every corner of the world, drawing on the food traditions of cultures from almost every continent, with ingredients shipped to us across the oceans and over thousands of miles. By one measurement, in fact, the ingredients of a single taco, all told, will have traveled sixty-four thousand miles from source to your stomach, forming an almost perfect antonym to the much-vaunted concept of localism.

In the instance of the taco, the foundation, the bread, is corn. Now, thousands of years ago, by some cosmic intuition that modern historians have yet to explain, nomadic peoples around the world came to understand that they could extract a basic diet from the grasses that they found growing all around them. In East Asia, that grass was rice. In Eurasia, it was wheat. In North America, it was corn. All three were domesticated at roughly the same time, so far as geneticists are now able to determine. All three provided the agricultural basis for the urban civilizations that would soon rise around fertile grain fields and paddies. And all three became staples of the world that spread far beyond their original homelands.

First domesticated in the Valley of Mexico, corn and the knowledge of how to grow it soon traveled into the Southwest, transmitted along river valleys and up mountain corridors until no culture in the region lacked for it. O'odham people in the river-laced valleys of what are now Tucson and Phoenix were growing it more than four thousand years ago. It arrived at other points in the Southwest at about the same time, fanning out in all directions from that southerly point of origin, and it has never lost its importance since.

As to the filling, it can be quite varied—for the taco is a versatile thing, and we can put lots of things on and in it and still call it a taco, much as we can use many different devices and words and still have a poem. A taco, like Gertrude Stein's rose, is a taco is a taco, very nearly a Platonic form as much as a food.

When people first came to the Southwest, at least twelve thousand years but perhaps much longer ago, they came to a region that looked far different than it does today, thanks to a generous, wet climate that resulted in plant- and animal-rich communities that were easy for the taking. When that climate turned arid, though, the land became less giving. When the Spanish arrived, well after the driest of these dry times, they brought new fillings, adding yet more diversity to that ancestral nosh. They brought cattle, animals domesticated out on the plains of Eurasia ten thousand years ago. They brought chickens, native to South and Southeast Asia and introduced to the ancient Mediterranean some twenty-five hundred years ago. They brought pigs, which the ancient Sumerians who lived in Mesopotamia—not far from where wheat was first domesticated—were keeping and eating five millennia ago.

Fillings attended to, we have toppings and condiments to add. Lettuce, for one, originally a wild green from the highlands of southwestern Asia and depicted on ancient Egyptian tombstones sixty-five hundred years old. Possibly some cabbage, a native of the Mediterranean. We can put radishes on top of our tacos, as is common in Mexico, eating a food that, according to the ancient historian Herodotus, was a favorite snack of the workers who built the pyramids along the Nile all those years ago. We can even stuff a few bean sprouts in there, honoring the cuisine of China, where mung and soya beans have been grown for thousands of years. Add cheese, tomatoes, avocado, pickled carrots, and any number of other ingredients, or add nothing else, and you still have an example of a food item that carries a passport with many stamps, that Platonic taco of dreams.

It's a mixed-up world, to be sure. One of the good ways in which it can be mixed up is in the things we find in our refrigerators. Look inside at the food you find there, and you'll see that what you eat every day is a blend of many traditions, cultures, and ethnicities. The taco alone is a multicultural wonder, and though we associate it with a single food tradition, it speaks to dozens. That is the story of the food of the Southwest, which is in turn a chapter, astonishingly rich and satisfyingly microcosmic, in the history of the food of the world. The taco is just one of its avatars, invented outside the region but mediated here and then transmitted to the rest of the world from this dusty entrepôt.

Inflow, outflow, invention, adaptation: That is the story I aim to tell in the pages that follow, with more about all these ingredients and the cultures that contributed them. You will be forgiven, though, if you wish to take a break now and go find a plate of tacos before moving forward.

Geographers have debated just where the Southwest begins and ends for generations. Some place Oklahoma in the region but disallow California. Some

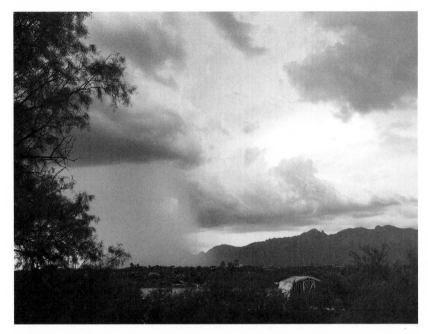

Sky, forest, mountain, grassland, and desert meet in a southwestern moment.

include California up to Big Sur or thereabouts, others Louisiana, in whole or up to the west bank of the Mississippi River. Some bring Utah into the fold, others not.

All these divisions have merits, especially those that give Louisiana outside the Florida Parishes a place in the region. From a strictly historical point of view, it would be easy enough to designate the Southwest as the region ceded to the United States after the Mexican War and the subsequent Gadsden Purchase, added to the Bourbon holdings incorporated under the terms of the Louisiana Purchase, but this is a little too generous, since it brings in all of Utah and even a little of Wyoming and Kansas.

In this book, the Southwest includes all of Texas and all of California, though California becomes somewhat less Southwestern when you go north of Milpas Street in Santa Barbara and its wonderful La Super-Rica Taqueria and becomes positively Northwestern by the time you hit Cape Mendocino. The region includes all of Arizona and New Mexico and southern Colorado up to the Gunnison River—in short, what geographers call the "core

Southwest." This has the unfortunate effect of ignoring much of Mexico, which we will include for reasons that will be obvious to anyone with a taste for the region's cuisine, and in any event it is unsatisfactory for another reason—namely, when we speak of the Southwest, we have it backward: Turn the map upside down, and you will see that we are really at the northwestern frontier of a world that stretches far south to the tropics and far beyond, ecologically to the Amazon and culturally to the tip of Tierra del Fuego.

For our purposes, the Southwest is anywhere Mexican influence is primary and of several generations' duration and where three cultures meet in roughly equal measure: Hispanic, Native American, and Anglo-American—European-descended peoples are known collectively as "Anglos" in the region. Many other cultures figure in the mix, and if today many components of the old mix are increasingly segregated everywhere but the kitchen, in the kitchen they still communicate easily with one another.

It is a huge region. California and Texas alone would swallow up most of Western Europe. It is geographically diverse. If we begin at California and work our way east, we leave a mild Mediterranean climate, climb tall mountains, and cross a vast rocky desert before even reaching the Colorado River. Arizona is a tangle of mountains and sandy valleys cut by mostly intermittent rivers; New Mexico is taller, colder, and mostly drier; Texas is a patchwork of desert, grasslands, plains, hills, and mountains that lead out onto another sea.

In this geography, high Colorado figures in the region as an extension of New Mexico, as do even small portions of western Oklahoma and Kansas. Nevada and Utah do not: They lie in a more Midwestern food tradition. There are culinary wonders to be had in the region, to be sure: Las Vegas is among the great eating cities of the West, and the pies of Mount Carmel Junction are not to be scorned. Even so, the tone of that region's cuisine favors the mildness of Iowa and not the fire of Yucatán, and thus we disqualify it.

And yet, Bettina Sandoval of the Indian Pueblo Cultural Center in Albuquerque pegs Southwestern food just right: "It's actually Mexican, Spanish, American, and Native cuisines combined." Put another way, then, the Southwest is anywhere that this is true—which allows us to claim portions of New York City, Washington, and Chicago in the bargain. Chicago, where Sandra Cisneros's food-filled novel *Caramelo*—its very title a lovely dish—is set, joined to ancestral land farther to the south and west, that syncretic place where breakfast is "a basket of *pan dulce*, Mexican sweet bread; hotcakes with honey; or steak; *frijoles* with fresh *cilantro*; *molletes*; or scrambled eggs with *chorizo*; eggs *a la mexicana* with tomato, onion, and *chile*; or *huevos rancheros*." And that's just the first meal of the day.

Put still another way, the Southwest is anywhere one can get a taco in which most of its ingredients can be found well within sixty-four thousand miles of the table. One of the best tacos I have ever eaten, in the company of the writer Luis Alberto Urrea in a fly-busy but spotlessly clean stand just across from the cathedral in Tijuana, was made by hand, with tortillas straight off the comal and pork that tasted as if it had been raised specially for our paper plates. The proprietor was a lively, lovely woman of early middle age who might as well have had six hands for all the dazzling dexterity she displayed, serving thirty or so hungry diners shouting in their orders a single taco or a dozen at a time and often for multiple rounds. Without writing a thing down, she remembered just what each diner had ordered, with a bill that arrived orally and that was correct down to the centavo. For all I know—and so I was told—she did not know how to read or write.

But the *maestra de tacos* certainly knew how to cook, doing well while doing much good in the world by keeping a demanding audience very happy indeed. I hope this book brings some of that same happiness in the reading.

I. Origins

They came hungry. They had traveled across ice, mountains, water, across years and thousands of miles to find new land where food was abundant—for where they had come from, with the shortsightedness so typical of our kind, they had hunted great beasts such as the mammoth, woolly rhinoceros, and steppe wisent to extinction or nearly so, many others to scarcity and rarity, creating the very conditions that would set a hunting people on the move to find more generous killing grounds.

Just when humans arrived in the Southwest is a matter of much conjecture—and considerable scholarly debate. When I was an undergraduate anthropology student in the mid-1970s, it was taken as a matter of near-religious certainty that the first humans appeared, having walked over the Bering land bridge, exactly ten thousand years before the present, or about 8000 BCE. They then fanned out across the North American continent, eventually finding their way to Panama and thence to South America in an orderly fashion.

Well, to evoke the rascals of the Firesign Theatre, everything we knew then was wrong. Our view is considerably complicated today, with some archaeologists maintaining that South America was settled before North America, with a newly discovered rock art site in Nevada dated to fourteen thousand years before the

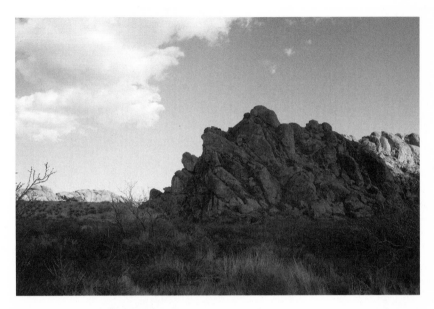

Hueco Tanks, in southwestern Texas, was an early site of human habitation in the Southwest.

present, with archaeological sites on the eastern edge of the core Southwest, along the Jornada del Muerto in south-central New Mexico, turning up evidence of human settlement as early as twenty-five thousand years before the present. In all the unsettlement over human settlement, the chronology has since been utterly rewritten, based in part on evidence that was controversial in its day but has become widely accepted, the paradigm shift in all its glory.

Archaeologist Richard MacNeish excavated two cave sites on the McGregor Firing Range, part of the vast Fort Bliss military reservation outside of El Paso, Texas. On these sites, not far from the Rio Grande, he found the flint-butchered bones of *Equus niobrensis*, a large horse that roamed the Great Plains until about thirty thousand years ago. Other bones—identified as the long-extinct Aztlan rabbit and extinct miniature Eohippus, or "dawn horse"—that have been found in association with human remains push the dates of occupation back to at least forty thousand years before the present, or about the same time the first aborigines crossed into Australia, itself then joined to Asia by another land bridge.

There is good reason to believe that other sites in the arid Southwest will extend the presence of humans in America much further back in antiquity. An old friend of mine, the archaeologist Julian Hayden, was convinced that evidence from shell middens—that is, heaps of discarded seashells, their contents eaten by humans—gave proof that humans were in the maritime desert of Baja California more than thirty-five thousand years ago and perhaps far earlier than that. Moreover, he believed, these people were of mixed ancestry, some from Cro-Magnon ethnic stock from Europe, others from northeastern Siberia, and others from Central and East Asia. Champions of a single-origin theory of the peopling of the Americas have rejected such arguments, but every day, it seems, news arrives to overthrow the old scholarship: recently, that there are some genetic linkages between western Eurasian peoples and Native Americans, pointing to mixed ancestry, and more recently still, that Australasian peoples may have constituted a wave of immigrants to the Americas twenty-three thousand years ago. Those dates conform nicely to recent archaeological work from a cave in what is now the Yukon Territory of Canada that has produced thousands of bones from caribou, horses, mammoths, and other animals in association with human tools dating to twenty-five thousand years ago, far earlier than the standard chronologies would allow.

All this is scholarly guesswork, but it is compelling, as is a recently published archaeological report that holds that, having left mainland Asia, the peoples who eventually arrived in North America spent more than ten thousand years in the country between, a place called Beringia after the great Arctic explorer Vitus Bering. They did so not because the scrubby lowlands were particularly scenic or even fruitful places to live but because great walls of glacial ice blocked most of the paths into the new continent—an obstacle that would disappear, some fifteen thousand years ago, thanks to a rapidly changing climate that would change the face of the world.

People do not often move out of sheer curiosity or for the pleasure of seeing new horizons. Instead, they are made to do so by thirst or hunger, by want or need.

Consider the Sahara: a vast, stony, sandy wasteland nearly the size of the continental United States, with only a few settlements of any size and a human population numbering in the few hundreds of thousands, a place whose name is a byword for the daunting and dangerous. Twelve thousand years ago, broad rivers crossed what is now the heart of that huge desert. Six great lakes, each larger than the states of New Jersey and Massachusetts combined, joined a network of streams and wetlands, and hundreds of smaller lakes and watercourses nourished a large human population of farmers and livestock herders—who, as we will see, contributed important elements to the food of the Southwest.

Some eight thousand years ago, a shift in climate heralded the onset of an arid trend that, with minor variations, has persisted in the Sahara today. Nearly all of the human and animal populations of the region's interior dispersed north and south to better-watered places, while those lakes and rivers dried up, leaving only a few scattered oases as reminders of their former expanse.

Thus it had ever been. What happened in the Sahara thousands of years ago happened millions of years ago, too. So severe was an arid period that began in the region of northern Africa six million years ago, for instance, that the Mediterranean Sea disappeared entirely. It was gone for nearly a million years. South and east of the present Sahara, in the Great Rift Valley of Kenya and Tanzania, a once-tropical landscape dried out. Where great forests had stood, savanna grasslands now emerged, dotted with scattered trees. Diverse species of ancestral great apes had once flourished, but their numbers thinned along with the trees, the landscape finally favoring creatures that were more adapted to life on the ground than in the branches.

There, in the parched rain shadow formed by the coastal highlands, the ancestors of modern humans emerged. The first of them walked on hands and feet, but in time—over millions of years, that is—they learned to walk upright, a critical adaptation. For one thing, by walking upright, those ancestral humans exposed less of their body mass to heat radiating upward from the ground in that sun-blasted landscape, protecting bodies and brains. For another, by learning to walk upright, they ushered in a mutation that straightened the larynx and enabled the production of meaningful new sounds—sounds that became language, the great gift of our kind.

Hominids slowly spread, turning up in places such as Java, the Caucasus, and Iberia, but their populations did not endure. Instead, eastern Africa remained the crucible of our species' evolution. There, about 180,000 years ago—give or take many thousands in either direction, for the chronology of human emergence is constantly being revised with new findings—the first

Homo sapiens developed. About a hundred thousand years ago, these Adams and Eves began to take their place in the fossil record outside of Africa.

Such dates match what climate historians have been learning about conditions in Africa during this time of evolution and adaptation. In the spring of 2008, a team of researchers examined a soil core sample pulled up from the bottom of Lake Malawi, at the southern end of the Great Rift Valley. Correlated with data taken from other sites, from plant pollen to fossil remains, the core sample records a series of megadroughts that occurred between 135,000 and 75,000 years ago, dates corresponding to the time at which recognizably modern humans began their migration out of torrid Africa. During that time, the team discovered, the water levels of Lake Malawi—which is today the world's ninth-largest inland body of water—dropped by nearly half a mile, which represents a loss of nearly 95 percent of the lake's volume before the drying trend began. Savannas turned to arid steppes and steppes to arid deserts in a series of environmental changes as severe as any in the record.

About seventy thousand years ago, though, the climate of the region began to grow wetter and more stable, with the lake regaining much of its former area. By that time, the human population of the Great Rift Valley was comparatively small, even as humans had spread beyond it, if in patterns that seem to defy logic.

The fossil record, for instance, shows ancestral humans hopscotching from East Africa to South Asia, then East Asia, and then Australia before winding their way to temperate Europe. Why? One theory suggests that the large-scale desertification of much of Africa at the time led humans to move to the coasts, foraging from the sea rather than the now-inhospitable land. Indeed, great piles of seashells in association with human remains along the Horn of Africa and Red Sea region point to a steady migration within sight of water but also to a point that archaeologists have long debated: Namely, that our prehistoric ancestors were probably very good sailors, capable of building oceangoing vessels to cross huge bodies of open water in their quest for greener pastures. That skill has implications for the peopling of the Americas.

Humans, of course, have another gift besides that of language, and that is a knack for adapting to conditions. Whereas, over millions of years, many animal species have disappeared because of an inability to adjust to environmental change—here the dinosaurs come to mind—humans have long seemed to thrive in the face of challenge. Adapting to abruptly changing ecological conditions has been a great engine in human evolution, propelling us into nearly every corner of the planet.

A comparatively modest warming period in what is now the Sahara some forty-five thousand years ago, for example, seems to have encouraged humans living along the North African coast to move eastward into the Arabian Peninsula, much of which was then a grassy prairie. There they merged with populations that had traveled upward from the Horn of Africa. Outliers of this new, Middle Eastern variety of *Homo sapiens*, which bears the chromosomal marker called M89, moved in one direction into Central Asia, in another into Europe.

The archaeological record, now supplemented by DNA studies across human populations ancient and modern, speaks to other migrations. Some ten thousand years ago, for instance, the Middle East became hotter and dryer than it had been during the Ice Age, anticipating the heating that would visit the Sahara comparatively soon in terms of geological time. Some of the people of the region moved inland to become pastoralists, following herds of goats, sheep, and cattle across the savanna; others became agriculturalists along the coasts, founding the world's first cities. That division between urban and nomadic still characterizes the region today.

Then there is the question of another great migration, noted by a genetic marker called M45. It joins the Upper Paleolithic peoples of Central Asia to the peoples of Europe and, across a vast sweep of time and space, to the peoples of North America, who arrived on the continent during another time of great climate change. Archaeologists and paleontologists will be absorbed for years to come in sorting out the facts and evidence but more in pondering the implications of that shared bit of chemical heritage.

All told, it took modern humans only the blink of an eye—forty thousand years, give or take a few score generations—to emerge from Africa and settle nearly every corner of the world. Climate change drove that great migration, just as climate change is affecting the movements of peoples today.

North and South America were the last continents on Earth to be peopled, and the process by which it happened is still a lively matter of scholarly debate. The best genetic evidence, from mitochondrial DNA, suggests that the earliest wave of migrants traveled along the coast of the eastern Pacific Ocean as far south as Tierra del Fuego, traveling by boat and land for generations, very much as those early migrants out of Africa traveled along the shore before moving inland as conditions permitted.

Other waves spread out over the interior of North America over a very long period of time. The first, as the linguist Joseph Greenberg has proposed, was made up of the speakers of ancestral American Indian languages such as the Uto-Aztecan tongues prevalent across much of the Southwest today. A second wave was made up of speakers of the ancestral Aleut and Eskimo languages, while a third wave brought speakers of what would become the Athabaskan languages, represented in the Southwest by Navajo and several Apachean groups.

This reconstruction of what has been called Paleoindian migration into the New World combines the study not of archaeological remains, which are scarce going back this far in time, but of historical linguistics, blood types, and dental patterns. We are on surer footing—and forgive the pun—with evidence that shows conclusively that people have been in the Southwest for a very long time. The oldest known human print in the Americas to date, a child's footprint dating to 13,000 BCE, was found in Chile—again giving credence to the theory that somehow settlement in South America preceded that to the north and adding a puzzling dimension to the history of the peopling of both continents.

In December 2013, archaeologists from Britain's Durham University announced that they had identified the oldest human footprints yet found in North America. Discovered in a place called Cuatro Ciénagas (Four Marshes) in the Mexican state of Chihuahua, which borders New Mexico and Texas, those footprints are more than 10,500 years old, predating the next-oldest set of footprints in North America by more than five thousand years.

When the first humans came here, they found a very different place from the one that we have today. Beginning about twenty-one thousand years ago, at the peak of the last major Ice Age, the Southwest was much wetter than it is today. The El Niño–La Niña oscillations brought regular westerly rains in from the Pacific, as much as forty inches a year in what is now the lower Sonoran Desert, or about what Iowa receives today. Much of that desert region was covered with a dense conifer and broadleaf forest, now characteristic only of the highlands. At the same time, most of Canada lay beneath a massive ice sheet, bounded to the south, along what is now the Pacific Northwest and High Plains, by a tundra zone resembling a polar desert. The deep cold that settled over the north had the effect of pushing the jet stream south, and storm pulses regularly arrived from the ocean, the phenomenon today called the Pineapple Express.

The Sonoran Desert, the homeland of what would become the Hohokam culture, was carpeted with ponderosa pine, alligator juniper, and other plants now found much higher up. The annual rainfall in the lowlands was more than forty inches, about the level Iowa now receives, and the mountains received nearly twice that amount. The land was the province of large animals that have since disappeared, many of which offered quite a larder for the Paleoindians, as archaeologists call the first peoples here. At Ventana Cave, Arizona, for instance, archaeologist Emil Haury catalogued evidence of their protein-rich diet: the bones of prairie dogs, otters, camels, short-faced bears, deer, badgers, wolves, jaguars, horses, and bison lay intermingled with scrapers, flint projectile points, and choppers.

We know about the early peoples of the region, thanks in part to rain, usually a welcome event in this dry land but sometimes too much of a good thing. On the night of August 27, 1908, a torrential rain began to fall on the small town of Folsom, New Mexico, in the northeastern corner of what was then a territory. The Cimarron River, which cut across a nearby mesa, soon overflowed its banks, and floodwaters gouged deep into the washes that fed into them. Folsom was destroyed, and seventeen people died. Surveying the damage, an African American cowboy named George McJunkin wandered into a place called Wild Horse Arroyo, deepened ten feet by the flood, and there found a pile of buffalo bones that were larger than those of modern bison. Moreover, he found a pile of intricately worked projectile points that moved the chronology of American Indians in the New World back ten thousand years and more. The news revolutionized the archaeological community, the rain having led to the discovery of the Folsom culture, as it is still known today.

That culture followed another tradition, the Clovis culture, which is better attested in the archaeological record. At Blackwater Draw, New Mexico, first excavated in 1929, spearheads were found that were longer and differently shaped from their Folsom kin. Those artifacts were associated with the remains of animals that would soon be hunted out, including the Columbian mammoth, smilodon, and dire wolf. Generations of people lived there, representatives of the Clovis, Folsom, Portales, and Archaic periods, the

Roast Mastodon

The instructions for roast mastodon are easy enough: Fell a mastodon, or a Columbian mammoth, or a gomphothere. Skin, butcher, fillet, and roast.

Granted, there are no mastodons or their kin to eat, and no right-thinking person would seek to substitute with their living cousin, the elephant. But consider that, thanks to advances in genomic technology, the possibility of bringing long-extinct creatures back to life is very real now—even dinosaurs, even if the majority of them should properly look more like to-scale chickens than giant Komodo dragons.

A combined South Korean and Russian research team is now following the noted paleontologist Björn Kurtén's wish to see mammoths brought back to life in the marshes of Siberia. Meanwhile, a team of Danish and Canadian researchers has announced the sequencing of DNA recovered from a kind of horse that lived in North America more than seven hundred thousand years ago. In theory, that horse is now a candidate for reintroduction.

Just because we can do so, should we? Jacob Bronowski, that wise scientist, long ago observed that our technology has always outpaced our ethical sense. Do we do any favors to a lost species by bringing it back into a world confronted with one environmental crisis after another? Will the passenger pigeon find the skies any friendlier today than they were when it disappeared a century ago?

Some say yes. Harvard geneticist George Church offers the possibility that those vaunted mammoths can themselves be agents of restoration for the taiga, even as the introduction of ancient genes into the modern gene pools of cheetahs, Tasmanian devils, and other species "could make them more tolerant of chemicals, heat, infection and drought."

Whatever the case, de-extinction, as this process of genetic restoration is called, is an attractive term in a time of massive extinction, and it heralds a debate that is likely to intensify in the coming years. Meanwhile, don't be surprised if soon a living mammoth appears on your television screen, a harbinger of returnees to come.

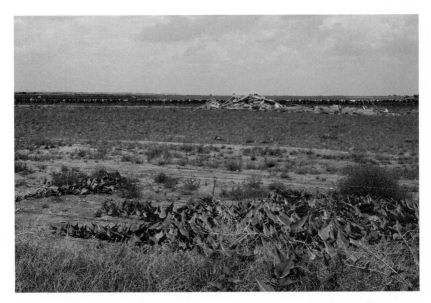

Ancient buffalo gourd flank more recently introduced cattle at Blackwater Draw, an ancient Clovis Culture site in northeastern New Mexico.

eventual ancestors of the Ancestral Puebloan and other peoples of the prehistoric Southwest.

Made of flint, a stone broadly distributed throughout the region, these spearheads, called Clovis points, are long and thin, shaped like an elm leaf. Even if their tips are broken, as many have been over the years, their rippled worked faces remain knife-sharp and strikingly lethal: those ripples produce a jagged cut that guarantees the hunter success, for if one of them strikes a target, the animal in question will soon bleed to death from its wounds, even if it is not killed outright.

Named for the New Mexico town where they were first discovered in 1936, these Clovis points mark an evolution of the migrant hunting peoples into accomplished technologists of stone. These Clovis peoples appear in the archaeological record at about thirteen thousand years ago—and so they are a beginning, if not absolutely *the* beginning, to our story. And it is no accident that the arrival of these Clovis peoples coincides with the last days on Earth for many animal species and populations.

We had long since adapted ourselves to cooking meat, having discovered fire and the energy it produces, and having gained huge advantages in terms of caloric energy from cooked foods in turn. "When our ancestors first obtained extra calories by cooking their food," writes biological anthropologist Richard Wrangham in *Catching Fire*, "they and their descendants passed on more genes than others of their species who ate raw. The result was a new evolutionary opportunity." That opportunity would, over millennia to come, lead people into every life zone and habitat, across ice and sand, and into a new world.

The Clovis hunters had another advantage: a knowledge of how to use dogs to help them in the hunt. The first humans in the Americas, the mitochondrial DNA of dogs suggests, arrived without these domesticated wolves, but somewhere along the way the Clovis people learned how to coexist with and, in a sense, co-opt the talents of these former competitors.

There were people in the Americas before the Clovis hunters, almost certainly, as we have seen. Recent evidence of their presence has been found as deep in the interior of the continent as the happily named Buttermilk Creek, a site near Austin, Texas, with remains dating to 15,500 years before the present. How they penetrated to the interior remains a matter of scholarly discussion, with the prevalent but not definitive view that they came down one of the narrow ice-free corridors on either side of the Canadian ice shield. Ancestral grizzly bears had traced the same route many years earlier, and they would have provided the greatest disincentive for the newly arrived humans, for these short-faced bears, as they were called, were highly efficient hunters of humans just as much as the hunters were efficient killers of mastodons and other megafauna, that is, animals weighing more than a hundred pounds.

In Beringia, that place of the ten-millennia-long layover, they would have found an abundance of megafauna: mammoths, bison, caribou, muskox, deer, dire wolves, smilodons (also known as saber-toothed cats), bears, yak, dall sheep, saiga antelope, moose, mountain lions. Smaller prey included squirrels, lynx, wild dogs, otters, ferrets, jaguars, lemmings, mice, voles, rabbits, wolverines, and foxes. Horses and camels, migrating between the continents, were prey long before they were beasts of burden elsewhere in the world. Pollen records, among other evidence, suggest that Beringia was mild and well watered about twenty thousand years ago, home to vast herds of ruminant animals that would have sustained a large human population as well as predators. With the advent of the Ice Age, though, the area became frigid and dry, inhospitable to those herds and, by extension, the animals that fed on them, forcing humans into the interior. Those predators would have created a formidable challenge for the hunters who dared follow the herds into the warmer country to the east and south—a challenge that led, in time, to the development of those lethal Clovis points and the culture that arose from them, a culture that made a commissary of the mammoth and that, absent the bears and tigers that fell to their spearpoints, became the reigning predators of the new land.

In the Southwest, the Columbian mammoth was their chief prey and the biggest animal any of the Ice Age people would ever see. In what is now the Mexican border state of Sonora, archaeological sites have revealed the remains of a cousin of the mammoth, the gomphothere, distinguished by its four tusks. More common in South America than north of the Isthmus of Panama, the gomphothere was thought to be extinct in the region until, just a few years ago, archaeologist Guadalupe Sanchez and her colleagues located gomphothere remains at a site in Sonora called El Fin del Mundo, the End of the World, as it certainly was for those unfortunate elephantine creatures. The work provides the first solid evidence that the Clovis hunters went after gomphotheres as well as their mammoth kin, and El Fin del Mundo is one of the oldest, and the southernmost, of all Clovis sites. Along with similar sites found in southern Texas, dating to 13,400 years before the present, El Fin del Mundo raises the intriguing possibility that the Clovis peoples might have originated in Mesoamerica and worked their way north, rather than the reverse—and that, as archaeologists have noted, has considerable implications in turn for the chronology of the peopling of the Americas.

Wherever they went, the Clovis peoples encountered a climate different from the one the Southwest experiences today. From the vantage point of San Gorgonio Pass, for instance, where towering mountains form the eastern border of the vast basin in which the metropolis lies, Los Angeles does not immediately seem a desert place. Sure, the Santa Ana winds howl, the hot air from the Mojave Desert spilling down to the sea and robbing the coastal breezes of their cool humidity. Sure, the television news warns of drought conditions not often seen in recorded history. Sure, prickly pears and date palms grow among the jacarandas and eucalyptus. But humans have been at work for generations to make a vast oasis of this once-arid region, carefully disguising much evidence of its desert heart, and on its best days the air of Los Angeles has a sweet mildness more befitting the Riviera than the Sahara.

From that same vantage point, it is hard to imagine that as recently as ten thousand years ago—and perhaps more recently still—glaciers once ground their way across the face of the San Gorgonio Mountains, the southern- and westernmost outpost of the last great Ice Age. Yet carve those glaciers did, lending a particularly sharp plunge to the western slope of San Gorgonio Peak, at 11,500 feet, the highest mountain in Southern California.

Those great sheets of glacial ice must have made quite a sight for the early Indian peoples who made their homes in the game-rich valley below. But the ice retreated into memory soon enough, disappearing as the earth warmed and the desert spread along the fringes of what was now a grassy, marshy plain, one that stretched from the mountains to the sea a hundred-odd miles in the distance. Over the millennia preceding the arrival of those Indian peoples, the huge basin saw a menagerie of animals that would disappear with the changing climate: mammoths, mastodons, dire wolves, ground sloth, ancestral horses and camels, and the saber-toothed tiger—all members of species that met their unfortunate end in the La Brea Tar Pits not far from present-day Hollywood.

Millennia before, at the northern fringe of what we are considering as the heartland Southwest, outside present-day Snowmass and Aspen, Colorado, a depression at an elevation of nine thousand feet filled with snowmelt during a period of regional warming. There mammoths, giant ground sloth, camels, horses, bears, and all sorts of other mammals gathered to drink— and some to die in the mud at the pool's banks. That these creatures were abundant at such high elevations as well as on the floor of what is now desert suggests both a temperate climate and a spectacularly rich fauna capable of sustaining large human populations. How large we cannot say, but we are certain that along with the humans, the short-faced bear, the American lion, and the saber-toothed cat—or smilodon—were competitors for game. They would have harvested great numbers of humans who were hunting the same things they were, and as a result, in what just as certainly was a coordinated effort involving hierarchy—someone concocting plans and assigning roles, someone else following them—human hunters took great pains to bring these creatures down wherever they were found.

When the Clovis culture and its lethal spearpoint developed—or arrived, depending on your interpretation—on the scene, numerous large-game species began to go extinct, along with those competing predators. A changing climate helped the hunters in their work, for as the deserts became deserts in the true sense of the word and the inland lakes and seas that abounded in places such as the present-day Salton Sea of California and the Rio Grande Valley of Texas and New Mexico began to dry up, these animals began to concentrate near available sources of water. Hunters had only to look for water to find game. In the valley of the San Pedro River near Sierra Vista, Arizona, for instance, the Murray Springs Clovis Site dates to about 11,000 BCE. At that spot, Clovis hunters attacked and killed a mammoth, a young adult female who fell about forty feet from a water hole that mammoths had dug in the riverside mud. The archaeologists who discovered and excavated the site found an intact Clovis spearpoint and three fragments with the remains, while nearby lay butchering tools and thousands of flint flakes, as well as a tool made of mammoth bone that was used to straighten spear shafts—the only tool of its kind ever discovered in the Americas. Hunters from the same culture also killed eleven bison here, members of an extinct Ice Age species. Blackwater Draw, one of the earliest known Clovis sites, shows similar evidence of prolific killing: the bones of Columbian mammoths, camels, horses, bison, smilodons, and dire wolves, among others.

We can say two things of those Clovis hunters: They liked to eat meat, and they didn't know when to stop. They followed herds until the herds were gone, killed elephants until there were no more elephants. But that, it seems, is the human way: Everywhere our kind has traveled, we have reduced the number and diversity of the animals that we have found. The late Quaternary megafaunal extinctions of ten thousand–odd years ago and the modern mass extinctions we are witnessing around the planet are all of an unhappy piece. Scientists at Aarhus University, in Denmark, recently completed a global analysis of that trajectory, tracking humans as they systematically removed species such as the rhinoceros and Eurasian elk from northern Europe, the mammoth from North America, the thylacine from Tasmania, and so forth. Perhaps counterintuitively, it is the continent from which that hungry migration first occurred, Africa, that remains the planet's only large region with a high diversity of mammals. But, says a Danish scientist, "The reason that many safaris target Africa is not because the continent is naturally abnormally rich in species of mammals. Instead it reflects that it's one of the only places where human activities have not yet wiped out most of the large animals."

The life of so-called primitive people, Thomas Hobbes famously—or infamously—remarked, is "nasty, brutish, and short." Half a century ago, anthropologist Marshall Sahlins decided to test this assertion by examining the relative fortunes of hunting and hunter-gatherer groups. He found that the traditional Xan people of the Kalahari Desert, to name just one of them, seldom worked more than four hours a day to support their families with the food and material goods they needed to sustain their idea of a happy existence. "The food quest is so successful that half the time the people do not know what to do with themselves," he noted, dubbing Hobbes's "brutish" peoples instead the "original affluent society." In the much less austere confines of the ancient Southwest, the Clovis hunters likely had it easier still. To be sure, hunting down one-ton bison and other megafauna was good for a workout—not just the killing, but the butchering and hauling would have required social coordination as well as physical strength, with bursts of hard work followed by periods of leisure and companionship.

There was other work to be done, too. There was, for example, the gathering of stones from which to make tools, or lithics, that flew straight and true, cut well, and could be used to make other tools: spears, arrows, axes, knives, hammers, and grinders. The ancient peoples, astute students of the land, would have gathered materials from sites that produced particularly good stone, such as Florida Mountain south of the Mimbres Valley of south-central New Mexico, where an ancient quarry yielded andesite, rhyolite, chert, quartzite, and obsidian. The Alibates Flint Quarries, located along the Canadian River in the far northern Texas Panhandle, was another prime site for high-quality toolmaking material, and there is evidence of human activity there stretching back thousands of years. As the Texas State Historical Association observes, "the working of Alibates flint could be characterized as one of the earliest and longest-lived industries in early America," since chipped stone taken from the site turns up in Clovis-era tools and was used by Native peoples until the nineteenth century, trading it across the continent: Panhandle sites show that the flint was traded for ceramics from the Rio Grande valley, obsidian from the Jemez Mountains in New Mexico, pipestone from Minnesota, and sea snail shells from the Pacific coast of California.

Making Salt

Salt is a naturally occurring mineral that is essential for human survival and often not easy to obtain. Peoples in deserts throughout the world traditionally traveled to salt sources, whether ancient lakebeds or the distant ocean, to acquire it.

A rule of thumb is that it takes five gallons of saltwater to make four cups of salt. This salt can be separated from the water by simmering—not boiling, but simmering—the water until it cooks down, then straining it through cloth or grass or else pouring it into a shallow pan and allowing the rest of the water to evaporate.

Any way you do it, it's a laborious process, which explains why the many varieties of salt available to us at high-end stores are so expensive. But once you see how cheap table salt is produced—there are places throughout the Southwest where this is done, including metropolitan Phoenix—you may not mind paying the premium.

In the same manner, the ancient peoples traded and traveled widely to procure salt, moving along an extensive network of trails leading to salt sources. Ancient people walked to the sea or deep into river canyons in search of it, as the ancestors of the Hopi people and their descendants traveled for salt to the junction of the Colorado and Little Colorado Rivers, to the Sipapu, a place where ancient stories say the human journey began.

A story that a cousin people of the Hopi, the Cochiti people of New Mexico's upper Rio Grande region, tell relates the travails of Old Salt Woman, who came to their pueblo and went from house to house looking for food, only to be sneered at and turned away. Angry, she led the children of the pueblo to a piñon tree and turned them into jays, squawking in shame and fear at their transformation from people to birds. She then went south along the river to Santo Domingo Pueblo, where the people fed her willingly and well. In thanks, she left them some of her body—salt, in other words—and then returned to her home at the ancient salt lakes that lie in the mountains of east-central New Mexico, near the present-day Salinas Pueblo Missions National Monument. Old Salt Woman is one of many female deities honored by Uto-Aztecan peoples, one of the best known of whom is the salt goddess of the Aztecs themselves, the guardian of the salt supply: She is depicted as having golden ears and wearing golden robes, a tunic in the shape of a wave, cotton sandals, a fishnet skirt, and, an imposing sight, a shimmering miter topped with a macaw feather.

The ancestors of the modern O'odham people of southern Arizona and northwestern Sonora traveled across *He'kugam vo:g*, "ancient trails," a phrase that means more than the physical path: The journey is a ceremony, the quest a sacrament, and the object of the journey across hundreds of miles a blessing. As they traveled, traditional O'odham sang songs marking the places they passed, mountains and rivers and desert valleys: as Andrew Darling and Barnaby Lewis of the Gila River Indian Community observe, "In a world without maps, a person who knows the songs is someone who not only knows where he or she is going, but more importantly, can recognize the dangers along the way."

We can conjecture that the Clovis people sang their way across the land, too. So ethnographic analogy suggests, since traveling peoples everywhere like to mark their voyages with song. We can conjecture that from time to time they fought for the salt as well, just as modern peoples have. The early Spanish settlers of El Paso, in the Rio Grande valley, traveled to the base of the Guadalupe Mountains to gather salt from dry lakes there, fighting Apaches to do so—Apaches who had fought other indigenous peoples for control of the resource. Centuries later, the same dry lakes would see conflict between two peoples and two systems of law: Following their law, the Spanish and later Mexicans of El Paso were able to make use of the salt freely, for it belonged to the king, and the king had generously given the salt to his people. Following their law, the Americans who came to rule the land after 1848 decreed that the salt instead belonged to the person or persons who owned the lakes. When the American who held the deed learned that Mexicans from Doña Ana County, New Mexico, were gathering salt at Lake Lucero, he ordered the sheriff to drive them away, resulting in an armed clash, in what history now knows as the El Paso Salt War.

In the main, though, the archaeological record suggests that salt was traded peaceably, as were many other goods. Over the passage of time, Clovis culture evolved into numerous traditions that archaeologists collectively call the Archaic culture. The time of abundant meat faded away as these cultures came to be at home in the Southwest, but the old journeys and the old ways continued, allowing the people to recognize where they were going—and where danger lay.

2. Native America

G iven enough time and will, we humans are adaptable creatures, capable of surviving and even flourishing in many
diverse environments and under many conditions. In that we
are like coyotes, which may explain why the Native peoples of
the Southwest hold their kinsman, *Canis latrans*, in such high
regard.

Here is one Coyote story, this one related by the Akimel
O'odham—the people of the flowing water, otherwise known
as Pima, who historically made their homes along the middle
Gila River and Salt River near the northernmost stretches of
the Sonoran Desert in central Arizona. Eagle, it seems, who
lived high in the sky, was annoyed because Coyote was so
painfully noisy all the time. Eagle reckoned that he would steal
Coyote's wife and give Coyote something to cry about. Turkey
Vulture saw Eagle carrying off Coyote's bride, and he told Coyote, "I know where your wife is. I'll tell you where she is and
take you there. But from now on, whenever you kill something,
you must always leave something for me." Coyote promised to
do as Turkey Vulture said, and Turkey Vulture flew into the
sky with Coyote on his back, finally gluing Coyote's eyes
together with mesquite pitch so that Coyote wouldn't become

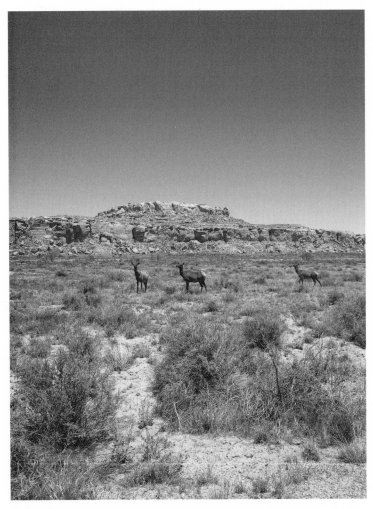

Mule deer at Chaco Canyon, New Mexico.

dizzy on looking down. When they arrived in the sky, Coyote was hungry—Coyote is always hungry—so he went from house to house, begging. Someone inside said, "Don't feed him. He lives far below us. Whenever I go down there to catch animals they chase me away." Coyote left again. He began to think he was going to die of hunger. Then he decided to steal something. He went to a house where no one was home and found a sack of cornmeal. He was about to eat when someone yelled at him, "Scat! Scat!"

Coyote ran away with the sack in his teeth. The cornmeal that Coyote scattered when he ran away can be seen up there now: the stars in the sky.

The Pleistocene megafauna, those creatures of a hundred pounds or more, had been pretty well played out across the Southwest by the end of the Clovis era, about twelve thousand years ago. It was a pyrrhic victory for the Clovis peoples, whose culture itself soon began to splinter into numerous smaller traditions that archaeologists have given various names, mostly with *archaic* or *paleo* affixed.

The loss of large game marked a profound change, but it did not mean that the people were forced into want. Instead, for many thousands of years, the ancient peoples of the Southwest learned to diversify. One way they did so was to broaden the sources of animal proteins. Now the bones of rabbits, mice, and other small mammals began to turn up in garbage middens, along with tortoise shells and the bones of small reptiles.

An important source of protein throughout Mesoamerica was the dog, which came to the North American continent at some point thousands of years after the earliest human migrants, probably arriving in the late Pleistocene. (That said, archaeologist William Doelle notes that "the first recognizable members of the dog family developed some forty million years ago in what is now southwestern Texas. So, with this lengthy family tree, dogs have a much deeper history in the Southwest than we humans do.") Mesoamericans such as the Olmec and Maya raised small hairless dogs for consumption, beginning about four thousand years ago. The Aztecs called the creature *Xoloitzcuintli*. Hernán Cortés, the Spanish conquistador, wrote of the many stalls given over in Aztec marketplaces for the sale of them, and so great was the demand for its meat that the wrinkly, small Xoloitzcuintli was on the road to extinction by the time Cortés made his notes. After the Spanish conquest, the eating of dog meat declined, but the Xoloitzcuintli still hovered on the edge of extinction until, in the 1940s, the Mexican artists Diego Rivera and Frida Kahlo helped bring the breed back and popularize it.

In the Southwest, the habit of eating dog meat did not catch on, as it did to both the south and the north. At one site in Sonora, archaeologist John Carpenter found the remains of more than thirty dogs buried among dead humans, which he interprets to mean that dogs were seen as being part of the community. In the more than four hundred roasting pits on the site, he adds, there has not been a single dog bone, which certainly would not have been the case deeper into Mesoamerica. Similarly, at Pueblo Grande, within sight of present-day Sky Harbor International Airport in Phoenix, Hohokam settlers buried fifteen dogs together. None showed butchering marks or signs of burning, though the presence of numerous dogs buried together has led archaeologists to speculate that they may have been buried alive with a powerful human to accompany him or her on the journey into the afterlife. That did not keep the prehistoric people of the region from occasionally eating coyotes, however, suggesting that they drew a distinction between coyotes and dogs. Faunal remains at one site included numerous coyotes, along with jackrabbits, squirrels, rodents, and deer.

A considerable amount of protein came from sources that are less palatable to us moderns, though—especially insects, which are being rediscovered today in some of Mexico City's finer restaurants, with the *chicatana*, or giant winged ant, recently selling for $225 a pound. Mexico, along with the borderland Southwest, boasts more than five hundred species of edible insects, more than any other country on Earth, and connoisseurs today are avid for such things as *ahuatle*, or water bug eggs, and *cumiles*, or stinkbugs, which, reports the *Washington Post*, "are prized for their powerful aniselike flavor and cinnamon finish." The squeamish are warned that, just as they probably were in the past, the stinkbugs are served live.

At a cave near a place called High Rolls, New Mexico, archaeologists found human coprolites—that is, fecal remains—with chewed bug parts evident throughout. High Rolls lies at the southernmost tip of the Sacramento Mountains above the broad grassland called Otero Mesa, near abundant perennial mountain streams full of trout. However, there are no signs at the site of fish consumption, which suggests that the ancient peoples had some sort of taboo avoidance. Steven Lentz, the director of the dig, speculates that the people there associated fish with the spirits of departed humans, a belief shared by other Native peoples in the region today. The people of High Rolls also consumed a great deal of ash, which helps settle a stomach bothered by parasites or diarrhea, suggesting that while the insect diet may have helped meet the people's protein needs, it also caused occasional distress.

In the mountains, those archaic hunters went after bighorn sheep. Down on the lowlands, they hunted bison, one of the rare megafaunal species to survive human activity until the nineteenth century. They were particularly successful, the faunal remains show, in bringing down pronghorn, using atlatls, or spear-throwers, to launch sharp darts at their prey.

Especially abundant at the site, which dates to about thirty-five hundred years before the present, are the bones of wild turkeys. Linguists have shown that the words for those birds and for agaves often traveled together, suggesting that they were incorporated into ancient diets at about the same time—and perhaps spread from the ancestral homeland of speakers of the hypothetical language called Proto Uto-Aztecan, the mother language of tongues ranging from Puebloan languages in the Rio Grande Valley to the Shoshonean languages spoken throughout the Great Basin to languages spoken as far west as the California coast (Luiseño) to eastern Texas (Comanche) and deep into Mexico (Nahuatl). Later sites across the Southwest show that the turkey was broadly domesticated, kept in pens or coops or allowed to roam freely around human settlements. At a Tewa Pueblo site near Santa Fe, archaeologists discovered evidence of a modestly scaled turkey industry involving hundreds of birds not just for meat and eggs but also for feathers woven into ceremonial blankets and clothing.

The Southwestern peoples' adaptation to place expressed its broadest genius in the use of plants. Ethnobotanists have estimated that across the borderlands region that defines the Southwestern heartland, those peoples collectively made use of twenty-four hundred to twenty-five hundred plant species—a very far cry from the two or three dozen that most modern Americans enjoy.

At the High Rolls cave site, located more than a mile in elevation in rugged but well-watered country, archaeologists found datura (Jimson weed), amaranth, tobacco, purslane, morning glory, dropseed grass, sunflower seed, feather grass, sotol, mesquite, yucca, and agave. Steven Lentz also noted a curiosity: His team excavated a yucca pod "stuffed with a mixture of goosefoot, pigweed, amaranth and other wild seeds." Lentz dubs this "the earliest breakfast burrito," which, of course, is exactly what the thing is, save that the diner was apparently in some hurry or else beset by some stomach ailment, since the burrito lay abandoned and half-eaten for centuries right where it was dropped.

Amaranth is an interesting case in point, a plant that traveled far from its Mesoamerican homeland long before Europeans arrived on the continent. Mediterranean amaranth, *Amaranthus cruentus*, a symbol of immortality in

Egypt and Greece, is botanically distinct from common American amaranth, *Amaranthus hypochondriachus*. By happy accident, however, the American amaranth, a native of Mexico and Central America, was also a symbol of immortality, especially to the Aztecs. When the Spanish conquistador Pedro de Alvarado arrived in the Aztec capital of Tenochtitlan, he discovered that its residents were fond of eating tamales filled with a paste made of amaranth seeds, a treat that honored the agricultural god Huitzilopochtli, granter of eternal life and the beneficiary of spectacular human sacrifices. Montezuma, Huitzilopochtli's earthly representative, received an annual tribute of two hundred thousand bushels of amaranth grain from the states that made up the Aztec empire. Alvarado puzzled over these strange facts and then went about the business of conquest elsewhere, but the Spanish governors who followed him outlawed amaranth cultivation in an effort to uproot this sometimes bloody form of worship.

They had a point, those Spanish, but their ban was hard to enforce. The Aztecs took its cultivation underground, so to speak, and kept the seed stock healthy over the generations so that amaranth grows in genetic diversity throughout Mexico's temperate zones, where it has been cultivated for at least seven thousand years.

Many Native American tribes well to the north of the Aztec heartland, the Tarahumara of Mexico and the Hopi of present-day Arizona among them, had also taken up amaranth cultivation and made the plant an integral part of their traditional diet. This was all to the good for those peoples, for amaranth produces protein-rich greens that can be cooked or eaten raw; alfalfa-like sprouts; and fine flour from its milled or ground seeds. It is something of a wonder plant: higher in calcium than beet greens, higher in protein than spinach, amaranth is rich in essential amino acids like threonine, valine, leucine, methionine, and especially lysine, an alpha amino acid that is prevalent in beef and chicken but less so as a plant protein and that is essential for humans. And as a source of protein, amaranth grain ranks higher than cow's milk, soybeans, and whole wheat—not bad for a plant that American farmers in the Southwest would dismiss with the scornful name pigweed.

Amaranth found a welcome home in the arid Southwest, for it is drought resistant, hardy, and adaptable to many environments, so much so that it has been introduced to the Middle East, Africa, and India, where it now ranks as a major crop.

Amaranth Pasta

Amaranth pasta beats wheat-flour pasta nutritionally, and it is not at all hard to make: Heat ⅓ cup amaranth seeds in a pan until they pop, just like popcorn. Grind the popped seeds in a blender; you should get about a cup of meal. Combine this meal with one cup of all-purpose flour, two eggs, and 5 tablespoons of water. Process the mixture as you would any other pasta dough. It takes only five or six minutes to cook the noodles in boiling water. Amaranth meal can also be used in cornbread, tamales, granola, and many other dishes.

Along the present western borderlands, in what is now Sonora, indigenous people cultivated a wild grass that looked like a shock of exuberant wheat. *Panicum sonorum*, or panic grass, produces abundant tiny seeds that cluster at the top of the plant. These seeds also contain high concentrations of lysine. The early farmers would not have known the precise chemistry, but clearly they recognized the value of the plant, for apparently it was widespread throughout the Pimería Alta and was extensively cultivated in Hohokam fields. Even so, by the twentieth century it was forgotten, last described growing near a Warihio Indian village in far eastern Sonora in the 1930s. Plant scientists rediscovered it there half a century later, a story that one of them, Barney Burns, recounted enthusiastically in an article for the *Seedhead News*, published by Native Seeds, a conservancy that now sells seeds through its mail order catalog.

The same is true of a tiny member of the sage family, chia, which takes its name from an Aztec word meaning "oily." *Salvia columbariae*, native to central Mexico and widely grown there, probably came into the desert Southwest in a trader's bag of seeds thousands of years ago. It came to be at home in many prehistoric cultures, providing seeds that are tiny in size but densely packed with nutrients. Mixed with ground meal, the mucilaginous plants added bulk to foods, somewhat like okra, and provided a quick source of energy all their own thanks to their rich store of omega–3 fatty acids. Rediscovered in recent years thanks to the ceramic "chia pet," the plant, which also contains abundant fiber, antioxidants, and potassium, has other virtues that would have been useful in thin times, including the fact that chia seeds can be kept for long periods without going rancid.

Coyote was hungry, and so he stole cornmeal, and the mess he made put the stars into the sky.

The Aztecs, rulers of the central Mexican heartland from which corn first sprang, told a different story from that Akimel O'odham just-so tale. The gods, it seems, were pondering what to eat when an ant happened to wander by, carrying a kernel of corn. A black ant followed, carrying a black kernel, and then a red ant with a red kernel. One by one the gods adopted the ants and their grains: turquoise, yellow, brown, white, red, purple, black, and every other color, now knowing what was good to eat.

But there was corn before there were Aztecs, at least as such. Its wild ancestor is very different from the fat, juicy-kerneled, thick-eared corn that we know, a spindly, utterly unlikely looking grass called *teosinte*. The ears of grain it produces are hard, the kernels fewer than a dozen, so far from its domesticated descendant, in fact, that when it was first described botanically, teosinte was thought to be a cousin not of corn but of rice.

It was thanks to the labors of a botanist named George Beadle, who later won a Nobel Prize for his work in plant genetics, that the kinship was proven in the laboratory. Not until years later was a human connection similarly proven. This came from an archaeological site in Mexico in which stone milling tools containing residue of this early maize were unearthed and dated to eighty-seven hundred years ago. The early farmers who tamed teosinte were themselves pioneering botanists, for it was through a program of close observation and selective breeding that, over time, they were able to encourage teosinte to give more generous yields of kernels in less formidable casings— over time being a point to emphasize, for the time required to coax something like the corn we know from that grassy progenitor was at least several hundred years, with the first cobs classifiable as modern *Zea mays* not appearing until about fifty-five hundred years ago. With the accompanying change in genetic structure, plant scientists have documented, the amino acid lysine in teosinte becomes an asparagine in corn, which in turn controls the size of the kernels and, not coincidentally, causes them to stay attached to the cob rather than scattering easily, as they do with teosinte.

So where do the Aztecs enter the picture? Only in that later DNA typing suggests that the particular strain of teosinte that gave rise to modern corn came from the Balsas River valley in southern Mexico, bordering what would later become the Aztec heartland. And the Aztec empire had yet to form

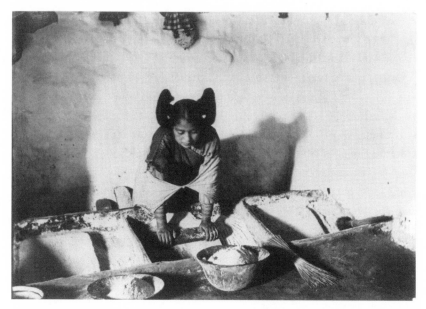

Hopi Indian girl grinding corn, about 1909. Courtesy of the Library of Congress.

when corn arrived in the Southwest more than five thousand years ago—again, in a chronology that is constantly being pushed backward with archaeological discoveries. For the moment, one baseline is the discovery of an ancestral hybrid of popcorn and pod corn at Bat Cave, a pre-Mogollon site in west-central New Mexico, dating to about fifty-six hundred years ago. Some ancestral group of people to the south, however, was responsible for a process that contains an Aztec element both linguistically and scientifically, namely nixtamalization, which involves soaking corn in a mineral lime or ash solution that makes it more easily digestible in the human gut, as well as easier to grind down into *masa*, or cornmeal. Though the scientific jury is out on the genealogy of that process, it seems fitting to credit it to the Aztecs, who built a great civilization on the basis of corn.

Hunting and gathering is typically an economy of just-in-time supply, with just enough food to see to the day and not many ways to store supplies away for another time. Agriculture operates on a different time scale and with a different theory. It presupposes that time is on the farmer's side, and it hinges on faith that there will be a surplus that requires managing so that there is food available in lean times of the year. It also demands staying in one place for at least part of the year, for a nomadic people cannot carry much surplus with it. With that settlement comes ceramics, for which nomadic peoples have little use but for which settled people soon develop a need, some durable way of keeping grain and other foods safe from rodents, insects, and the elements. Find ceramics at a site, and you can be sure that the people who made the pottery intended to stay—though whether the fates would conspire to allow them to do so was another matter. Settling down into an agricultural civilization brings with it bureaucracy, crime, epidemic diseases, and other drawbacks, but it also allows humans such things as the specialized division of labor, schools and libraries, and other good things in the trade-off. In the case of the Aztecs, corn allowed them to build pyramids, ball courts, great canal systems, luxurious palaces, and even an empire that would eventually dominate much of central Mexico for generations and whose influence was felt even in the remotest corners of the Southwest.

As with agaves and turkeys, it appears that the people who spread the cultivation of corn in the prehistoric Southwest were speakers of the protolanguage that would evolve into the Uto-Aztecan family of languages—and more specifically, suggests the eminent linguist Jane Hill, the northern branch of that protolanguage, which then loaned words for corn to the neighboring Kiowa-Tanoan languages spoken in the upper Rio Grande Valley and out on the plains of Texas. Just how this transmission occurred is a matter, as ever, of scholarly conjecture. One view is that some outlier group of hunter-gatherers in the upper Gila River drainage, which joins geologically to the Sierra Madrean mountain complex stretching deep into Mexico, came into contact with maize cultivators to the south and, after learning their agricultural arts, brought maize farming home with them. But plenty of signs of what archaeologists mildly call "discontinuities" turn up in the archaeological record, too, which collectively suggest the possibility of migration and outright invasion of what is now the Southwest from some southerly point of origin. For example, archaeologist Daniel Matson has shown that the earliest Ancestral Puebloan peoples on Cedar Mesa in southeastern Utah point to two lineages, one, called Eastern Basketmaker II, showing continuity with the archaic cultures of the region and the other, called Western Basketmaker II, showing strong connections to Mesoamerica. He suggests that the eastern branch borrowed maize cultivation from the western about five thousand years ago, which fits with a larger regional view of cultural contact. The Plains people loaned the Uto-Aztecans their word for bison, so that contact was a two-way affair.

The argument continues when it comes to the Hohokam culture of southern and central Arizona, the first settled agricultural civilization in the Southwest. For decades, archaeologists have debated whether the Hohokam were a people who migrated northward from Mesoamerica and settled among the ancestors of the O'odham or whether they were in the area all along and benefited from trade with Mesoamerican neighbors. Archaeologists who hold to the second position can point to the figure of Kokopelli as indirect evidence, for though sometimes interpreted as a beetle (and sometimes as an extraterrestrial being), the iconographic rock art figure nicely serves as the symbol for a wandering peddler from down in the Valley of Mexico who roamed the continent with a basket on his back full of things to trade, including seeds. It may be that a hybrid explanation best serves, for then as now the Southwest was the meeting place of many cultures and peoples, some just passing through, some staying to enjoy the view.

This was certainly true of Chaco Canyon, the preeminent city of the ancient Southwest. Located in northern New Mexico, with outlier settlements extending into Colorado and Arizona and even out onto the plains, it was occupied for hundreds of years. Like any city, it depended on resources drawn from the surrounding region—and such resources are often controlled at the point of a spear, suggesting that, like the Aztecs, the Ancestral Puebloan people of Chaco were able to field a formidable army.

If you have visited Chaco Canyon, then you know that the washboard dirt road that leads into the national monument from the north, the best of a couple of possible approaches, is a sort of nondescript experience, if a kidney-rattling and dusty one: You bounce around for an hour, then round a bend, pass a parking lot and campground to the visitor center, and then—and only then—begin to make out the remains of what was once a splendid city. But back up and imagine that you are a traveler from the hinterland, voyaging day after day on foot to reach this place a thousand years ago: A trail leads you atop a sandstone mesa, and from its top you stand astonished—exactly the effect its builders intended—as you look down at the largest, most resplendent city you have ever seen. Its walls are straight and long, its towers tall, its multistoried buildings neatly whitewashed, its plazas full of people, all of which unfolds as you descend a grand staircase into the heart of the city. Even in ruins, it is spectacular, with its intricate stonework and radiating avenues.

To build that great city required extraordinary resources, including a quarter of a million trees brought somehow from mountains more than fifty miles away—a mystery, as with the great Hohokam pueblos along the Gila River, given that the ancient Southwesterners did not know the wheel and had no pack animals. Even so, Chaco is served by great roads from which all kinds of trade goods came in from all over the Southwest: copper bells and tropical birds from far south in Mexico, bison horn from the plains, turquoise from distant mines—and from everywhere, all those supplies of corn, enough to feed thousands of urbanites.

A dozen years ago, I sat drinking coffee at four in the morning at a New York café across the street from Penn Station and watching the people come and go in a place as busy as any anthill. The wait staff were from the Balkans, the cashier from Russia, the cooks from Mexico and Central America, the clientele on that cold early morning from everywhere in the world, and as I watched plates of beef and eggs and ham and pancakes and endless pots of java pass by my field of vision, I had a reverie about—well, about Chaco Canyon, back home, and all the many-pathed trails and networks that brought food to that great city, just as a spider web of trade routes brought my breakfast to me that day. Making the choice to settle down was not easy for those early people, almost certainly, and entering that chain of supply and demand may not have been entirely or even in the least bit voluntary.

From the hands of those ancestors, corn has proved to be one of the economically most important crops the world has known. In the United States in 2010, it grew on a staggering eighty-six million acres of land in a yield surpassing twelve billion bushels. NASA scientists not long ago took satellite photographs measuring photosynthetic activity around the world showing that the Midwest at the height of corn-growing season is the biologically busiest part of the planet. That is a botanical success story that begins with a slender blade of grass thousands of years ago, a blade of grass that would change the world—a blade that at first produced ears of corn so small that, archaeologists believe, the ancient peoples did not eat them typewriter-style, as we do, but instead sucked on the cobs to extract what sugar they could from them, as if eating a weedy lollipop.

On an early spring day in 1536, four skeletal figures, dressed in tattered animal skins, turned up at the gate of a ranch in Sonora, where a guard challenged them. They answered in Spanish, the leader later recalling that he had despaired of ever seeing Christians apart from his companions—one of whom was a Muslim—again. Álvar Núñez Cabeza de Vaca had just turned forty-four. His companions were Andrés Dorantes de Carranza and Alonso de Castillo Maldonado, accompanied by Dorantes's servant, a manumitted slave called Estevánico, who, though called Moorish, was of black African ancestry and thus among the first Africans in North America. They had been shipwrecked off the coast of Texas, near the mouth of the Brazos River, eight years earlier. Their number had been three hundred or more when they were tossed up on the shore of the island they called Malhado, or Bad Luck. Now it was just them.

Cabeza de Vaca made careful mental notes of the geography they passed as the quartet walked across the continent, recording rivers, mountains, and prairies. He observed that about a hundred miles away from the coast, the Indian peoples he met consumed the fruits of prickly pear cacti, which he called *tunas*, promising the travelers that "we would eat many and would drink their juice and would have our bellies very big and would be very contented and happy and without any hunger"—or so he wrote, telegraphically, in his memoir, *Naufragios* (*Shipwrecks*). Moreover, he observed, the people closer to the coast made extensive use of the pecan trees that grew in profusion up the valleys of the San Antonio and Guadalupe Rivers, while those farther inland were fond of what he called *mesquiquez*, "a fruit that when it is on the tree very bitter and is like a carob bean and is eaten with earth and with this it is sweet and good to eat." The Indians, he added, pounded these beans with sturdy maces in a pit then made a kind of spongy bread of the dusty flour, emerging from the feast "with their bellies very big."

Cabeza de Vaca also observed that the peoples along the way traveled far to hunt deer, pronghorn, and especially bison, crossing into far distant territories where, he confided, there lay seven fabulous adjoining cities made entirely of gold. Their name, he said, was Cíbola.

Cabeza de Vaca soon ran into trouble with the ever-busy Inquisition, since he claimed to have enacted a few miracles along the way, and he was returned to Spain. His stories of gold continued to excite the Spanish imagination after his departure, but the realities he recorded were of more immediate practical value. Almost every Indian nation he encountered grew corn in enough quantities to offer it for trade, for instance, and few were seriously in want. Mesquite, widespread across the Southwest then as now, was one reason: The indigenous peoples who knew the tree also knew the protein-rich flour that could be made from the seeds. "From this a cake was made and either dried in the sun or baked," writes the pioneering botanist Edmund Jaeger, who recorded its use among numerous peoples who lived along the lower Colorado River. "Sometimes the Indians soaked the flour in water to make atole, a gruel-like sweet drink. If the infusion was allowed to ferment it resulted in an intoxicating drink of considerable alcoholic content."

In the eastern stretches of the region and into the South and the Mississippi Valley, the pecan had similar importance. Archaeologists have discovered pecans in association with human settlements dating as far back as 6700 BCE, almost to the time that the first farmers were experimenting with teosinte. Although the Native peoples did not tend orchards as such, there is considerable evidence that they extended the range of the tree and otherwise domesticated it—though never so far and so much as the industrial growers of pecan trees would in the twentieth century. So abundant were the groves near the southern Texas coast that the Spanish explorers who arrived there in the years following Cabeza de Vaca's passage called one broad stream Rio de Nueces, the River of Nuts.

In much of the Southwest, pinyon nuts, growing from a scrubby coniferous tree in the high desert, were important in the indigenous diet. The nut is rich in fats and carbohydrates, stores well, is easy to harvest, and is usually abundant, making it a boon for those people who knew it. Pinyon harvesting time afforded the opportunity for people to gather in late summer or fall, meeting distant family members and exchanging news while gathering nuts, using spliced willow poles to knock the cones from the trees, then carrying them to roasting pits that were a feature of permanent harvesting camps, at which archaeologists have found stacked grinding stones called *manos* and *metates*, set aside to serve subsequent harvests, in excavations dating back several thousand years. Pinyon nuts can be eaten raw or lightly roasted, but, like mesquite beans, they often found their way into various dishes of flour and gruel. Anthropologist Margaret Wheat notes that the Paiutes left pinyon paste out in cold weather to make a kind of ice cream, a favorite of young and old alike.

Here and there throughout the Southwest, but particularly in western California, oaks provided acorns that in turn provided meal. The Tongva, Maidu, and other peoples of the Pacific coast particularly prized black oak and canyon oak, while the Maidu, who lived in higher and more forested terrain, counted twelve kinds of acorns and related tales of the trees they came from, such as one about the tan, golden, and black acorn maidens who, at the beginning of time, were fearful that humans would find and devour them but eventually resolved themselves to that fate, only to find that only a few kinds of oaks lent themselves to the task, the plainer ones being more useful than the more beautiful.

Only a few kinds of people, conversely, made use of the agarita, sometimes called agarito or algerita, an evergreen shrub harvested by several peoples in what is now western Texas. The berries, rich in alkaloids, are bitterly astringent, and many peoples used them for medicinal purposes as laxatives or poultices. Some people, such as the Mescalero Apache, reportedly ate the fruit fresh off the bush, but this might serve to illustrate their legendary toughness, if not the old saw that much of the world's cuisine is at heart based on a dare.

One of the defining plants of the Sonoran Desert is the great columnar cactus called the saguaro (*Carnegiea gigantea*), which is central to the traditional agriculture of the desert peoples, the O'odham. *Hahshani bahithag mashath* ("the moon of the saguaro cactus fruit") is what the Tohono O'odham (the People of the Stony Ground or Desert People) call June, the onset of torrid summer, when the hunger and cold of winter and the dryness of spring give way to a new and more plentiful season. It is then that the saguaro brings forth a date-sized fruit that is both tart and sweet, which the O'odham then gather, knocking the fruits down from the top of the plant with a long pole called the *guiput*, laboring in the uncompromisingly hot sun. And once having done so, the Desert People make the rain come: The height of the harvest coincides with the feast day of St. John the Baptist on June 24, when, local tradition holds, the first monsoon clouds begin to swell up on the southern horizon. The O'odham gather the fruit to eat fresh from its host—it tastes something like a cross between a cucumber and a sweet watermelon—and to make a fast-fermented wine, *nawait*, that they use to invoke the summer rain. Anthropologists call the process "sympathetic magic": by the traditional formula, an adult will drink enough of the slightly acrid wine to induce vomiting.

Spilling from mouth to ground, the discharged wine encourages the rain to follow its lead, to pour from the clouds to the dry desert below. In this time, the children sing rain songs, lovely invocations for the clouds to come and bestow their blessings. So it is each June, this moon of the saguaro cactus fruit, when wine is made, the clouds are called up with ceremonial vomit, and the Tohono O'odham sing in the quiet corners of the desert. Poet and linguist Ofelia Zepeda offers a translation of one song:

Here you dropped it upon my land
And with that my land was sprinkled
with water and was finished.

Thus watered—and though a desert in every sense, it is the wettest in the world—the Sonoran Desert alone harbors some twenty-five hundred plant species, including three hundred species of cacti. Among them is the stately saguaro, which, strange to say, is a cousin many times removed of spinach.

Cuisine based on a dare, or so, to a squeamish diner, huitlacoche might seem. The even less sonorous name, corn smut, suggests that something unpleasant is afoot—and hold the word *foot* in mind, since the smell of huitlacoche can be suggestive of old socks. The fungus *Ustiago maydis* produces galls in corn, something akin to boils or even tumors in humans, mostly taking the place of normal kernels. Huitlacoche is rich in protein and lysine, which ordinary corn does not have. It is worth noting that ancient farmers prized huitlacoche for exactly this nutritious boost, while modern botanists observe that the fungus is often found in association with healthy and biodiverse plantings of corn—since, as might be expected, modern industrial genetically modified varieties do not provide suitable hosts.

Everything old is new again. Though huitlacoche has never gone away in traditional diets, trendy diners have been rediscovering it in Mexico City and even Paris, where it is marketed as "Aztec caviar" or "Mexican truffles." The few American menus where it appears have so far retained the original

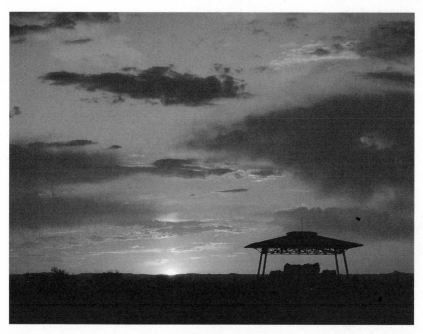

A winter sunrise over Casa Grande Ruins National Monument, Arizona.

Nahuatl name, although I have seen a few instances of "corn truffles," a nice euphemism that steers clear of false advertising while masking any ickiness. Huitlacoche, cooked with onions and queso blanco, is wonderful served with corn tortillas and amaranth greens.

If corn is one pillar of the ancient Southwestern diet, then beans are a second, and squash a third—the Three Sisters of Iroquois legend, having traveled thousands of miles from their Mesoamerican homeland. New World beans of the genus *Phaseolus* number about 125 species. Among them are the kidney bean, first domesticated on the Mexican plateau and present in the Southwest for millennia, and the tepary bean, a staple of indigenous diets across the region. Runner beans probably come from farther south in Mexico but have long enjoyed a similar reach across the Southwest. Hopi farmers reportedly discovered viable seeds in an ancient cave settlement and began to grow them in the 1940s, saying that the beans had the consistency and taste of mashed potatoes.

The sturdy lima bean was also a regional favorite. Many Native peoples, it is said, relied on beans when game was scarce and made out just fine, especially when corn was available, since corn and beans provide complementary proteins: beans lack cysteine and methionine, corn lacks lysine and tryptophan, but they complete each other nutritionally. Since beans store well, those Hopi farmers were not alone in keeping a healthy, diverse seed bank going, and modern gardeners have many ancient varieties to choose from, including the so-called Anasazi bean widely reintroduced from New Mexico in the 1980s and a number of delicious varieties sold by Native Seeds and other ethnobotanically minded growers. One in particular that Native Seeds has been working to reintroduce is the jack bean (*Canavalia ensiformis*), which appears in the archaeological record about fourteen hundred years ago but fell out of favor decades ago, last documented growing in Akimel O'odham fields in Sacaton, Arizona, in 1938. Drought resistant and with a pod that can grow to a foot in length, the bean is now being grown in gardens throughout the region.

First domesticated in central Mexico in about 7000 BCE, squash, along with other gourds, have been grown in the Southwest for millennia. When Mormon settlers came to the banks of the Gila and Salt Rivers in central Arizona in the 1860s, in fact, they gave their new towns religiously resonant names like Nephi and Lehi, which later became Tempe and Mesa, but called what is now the site of downtown Phoenix Pumpkinville, after the wild gourds that grew along the abandoned Hohokam canals. I prefer that name but so far have not been able to persuade the city fathers to adopt it anew so that we can cheer the Pumpkinville Suns on to victory.

Though essential in the Southwestern larder, another food plant has traveled somewhat less widely than corn, squash, and beans—at least until recently. *Capsicum annuum* and other species of chile peppers, numbering about thirty in all, are native to Mesoamerica and the northern Andean foothills, and they have been widely grown and traded throughout that region and into the Southwest for millennia, with the earliest evidence of cultivation dating to more than nine thousand years before the present. One of the oldest known sites for chile production lies in Tamaulipas, the Mexican state bordering southernmost Texas, which suggests (but does not prove) that cultivation traveled along the Gulf coast. The linguistic evidence in turn suggests that the Kiowa-Tanoan peoples of the Texas plains had chile for hundreds of

Roasting Chiles

In their raw form, chile peppers are encased in a skin that, while satisfyingly crunchy, is a chore to get through. Roasting the peppers separates the chile from the skin and caramelizes the sugars within them, adding flavor to an already flavorful food.

An early inhabitant of the Southwest might have used heated stones as an oven, or else cooked the peppers over open flame. Roasting over fire is the most pleasing way of approaching the task, to be sure: Place the peppers on a grill over charcoal or fuelwood and, with long tongs, turn them frequently to prevent the peppers from burning. You can also cook the chiles in a hot oven or broiler set at 400 degrees for a few minutes; cook them on a mesh frame over a burner on the stove; or even steam them in a microwave-safe dish in a microwave oven.

When peeling the skin, be wary of getting capsicum in your eyes or inside your nose. It helps to do this work in a sink under running water. Wear rubber gloves, and don't touch your face while doing so. As an added precaution, wear safety goggles—it nicely completes the mad scientist look. Use a sharp knife or vegetable peeler to remove any clinging skin. The peppers can be frozen in plastic freezer bags or containers for a year, until the next harvest.

years before it was grown in the Sonoran Desert, again pointing to an east-to-west transmission across the region.

Like tobacco, eggplant, potatoes, and tomatoes, all of which came into the Southwest later, chiles are members of the nightshade family, poisonous to some degree or another in their ancestral forms but long since bred for safe consumption. Many chile varieties awaited Spanish colonization to travel north out of Mexico, but the native chiltepin, reckoned to be one of those ancestral varieties, was widespread. Reportedly, the Tarahumara people of the mountainous country of the central Chihuahuan Desert held that anyone who could not eat chile was a sorcerer, and that seems about right. Whatever the case, though psychologists number being "bitten" by chiles—*capsicum* comes from the ancient Greek word for bite—among the so-called negative events the world has to offer us, they also note that humans are the only known species to deliberately seek out such experiences. Incidentally, the ability to detect capsaicin, the active biting ingredient in chiles, is a human universal, and people across the human spectrum are able to tolerate chiles physiologically. What makes some people feel as if they are on fire while others feel a pleasant warmth is more cultural than biological, which will do nothing at all to prevent your reaching for that glass of quenching water (or, better, milk) when you get hold of a red-hot specimen from Hatch or some other fine Southwestern terroir. Just know that when you do, you are doing your body a world of good, for chiles are rich in vitamins A, B, C, and E; betacarotene and other antioxidants; and iron and potassium. They block the absorption of cholesterol while boosting metabolic rates otherwise, making them a great diet aid, and they have been widely used to help alleviate pain thanks to their role in helping the body release endorphins.

Corn, beans, squash, chiles, the four essential plants in the cuisine of the Southwest, along with various animal proteins. Put them together, and you have the makings of an adventurous, nonrepetitive, even exciting cuisine. Consider a feast that Bernardino de Sahagún, the Spanish chronicler and Franciscan friar, partook of in Mexico City in about 1530, which offered

> turkey with a sauce of small chilis, tomatoes, and ground squash seeds; turkey with red chilis; turkey with yellow chilis; turkey with green chilis; venison sprinkled with seeds; hare with sauce; rabbit with sauce; meat stewed with maize, red chili, tomatoes, and ground squash seeds; venison with red chili, tomatoes, and ground squash seeds; birds with toasted maize; small birds; dried duck; . . . white fish with yellow chili; grey fish with red chili, tomatoes, and ground squash seeds; frog with green chilis; newt with yellow chili; tadpoles with small chilis; small fish with small chilis; winged ants with savory herbs; locusts with chi'a; maguey grubs with a sauce of small chilis; lobster with red chili, tomatoes, and ground squash seeds; sardines with red chili, tomatoes, and ground squash seeds; large fish with the same; a sauce of unripened plums with white fish . . . Tuna cactus fruit of many hues . . . tamales made of maize flowers with ground amaranth seed and cherries added; tortillas of green maize or of tender maize; tamales stuffed with amaranth greens; tortillas made with honey, or with tuna cactus fruit; tamales made with honey . . . gophers with sauce; hot maize gruel of many kinds; maize gruel with honey, with chili and honey, with yellow

chili; white, thick gruel with a scattering of maize grains; sour, white maize gruel; sour, red maize gruel with fruit and chili.

No Southwestern board after Chaco Canyon could have competed with that. Still, across the Southwest, Native peoples enjoyed a diet that, with many local variations, might have included corn gruel, tamales, beans, iguana and snake, deer, insects and worms, spirulina, mesquite flour, fruit, honey, agaves, squashes, and many other kinds of seeds and plants, to say nothing of various alcoholic beverages. People living near streams and rivers might have enjoyed fish, while those along the coast of the Gulf of California, as the biologist Richard Brusca has enumerated, "were feeding on shellfish, finfish, crabs, and sea turtles from coastal lagoons and the open coast, although they also captured some terrestrial reptiles, mammals, and birds." Peoples along the Gulf of Mexico enjoyed a similar bounty, though, to trust Cabeza de Vaca, their reliance on gathering disinclined many of them to agriculture.

Put these all together, and you have a storied and varied food tradition that extends back many thousands of years. Or, better, food traditions, for in many places, such as Bat Cave up on the Mogollon Rim and High Rolls in the Sacramento Mountains, as well as along the Gulf of Mexico, the old ways of hunting and gathering are attested side by side with the revolutionary way of life introduced by farming. That new way of life came in on many desert trails. Botanical detectives studying the DNA of corn have identified a highland route following the Sierra Madre and separate trails following the lowland coasts, with a meeting place of both zones evident at a fifty-five-hundred-year-old rock shelter in the Mexican state of Nuevo León, not far from the place where the Rio Grande meets the sea and the trail of Cabeza de Vaca, where corn, beans, squash, chiles, and other plant remains were found alongside the bones of lizards, birds, and small mammals. That diversity speaks to the development of the milpa system of farming, in which crops were mixed and complementary, often numbering a dozen or more kinds of plants.

The people there may have had to work for their daily bread, but they did not want, and they stayed at that rock shelter for generation on generation, building hearths and altars, meeting spaces, and houses on the rocky slopes outside the cave. It may not have been paradise, of course, at least for the women: Nixtamalization was followed by hour on hour of grinding wet corn with rock mills by hand, after all—from four to eight hours each and every day, since nixtamalized dough begins to ferment within twenty-four hours, making it something altogether different. But it sufficed, and agriculture was central to a life free of the old cycles of feast and famine. So central was corn to that tradition that the Navajo, who came into the Southwest at about the time the power of the Ancestral Puebloan builders of Chaco had declined completely, linked corn to the very process of creation. Washington Matthews, the Irish-born chronicler of Navajo ways, recorded at the end of the nineteenth century a Navajo story about the first people to emerge in this new land:

> Ordered by the creator gods to wash, since they had acquired a
> certain tang on the long journey, these first people bathed themselves
> thoroughly on the twelfth day, then dried themselves with cornmeal,
> the women with yellow cornmeal and the men with white. The gods
> were pleased, so much so that they then made new people, First Man
> and First Woman, out of white and yellow corn; they then filled the
> land with people who, remembering their origins in the grass, have
> cultivated corn ever since.

Let us close not with that but, appropriately, with dessert. *Chocolatl*, as the Aztecs called it, is a spice derived from the cocoa bean, a stimulant with an enormous freight of symbolism attached to it. Archaeologists have dated the consumption of chocolate to less than four thousand years ago, though it is likely that its history stretches into the more distant past. The basis of mole, the chocolate- and chile-laced sauces served with turkey and other fowl, chocolate would have served the role of a spice or condiment in ordinary cuisine—though no connoisseur would consider a diet involving chocolate to be ordinary.

Curiously, evidence of the earliest use of chocolate in the Southwest, dating to about twelve hundred years ago, comes from a humble site near what is now Canyonlands National Park, in southeastern Utah. One might have thought that the substance would have been reserved for the elite of Chaco Canyon and not a desert pithouse far to the north and out of the way even then. It may have served a ceremonial function so far from its Mesoamerican homeland, where chocolate most definitely was a treat reserved for the powerful.

To name one of those elites, accustomed to fabulous feasts, the Emperor Montezuma, it is said, drank fifty cups of chocolate a day. We have that information from the Spanish conquistador Hernán Cortés, who took careful notes wherever he went and whose arrival initiated a new period in the formation of Southwestern cuisine.

3. **Entradas**

On October 14, 1492, Carib Indians paddled out to a newly arrived caravel in a Bahamian harbor, bringing what its captain, Christopher Columbus, described only as "various kinds of food," including bread made of corn and fish of a sort the Spanish crew had not seen before. The next day, Columbus offered wheat bread and honey to his visitors, thus initiating what has since been called the "Columbian exchange" of food plants and other goods among the known continents.

That exchange, from the European point of view, was utterly transformative. To conceive of the depth of how it changed the European diet, we have only to imagine life without pizza or spaghetti, grilled steak without corn on the cob, hamburger without french fries, french fries without catsup, a horrific world without chocolate ice cream, coffee, and pumpkin pie at Thanksgiving.

The diet of the Old World before the European arrival in the Americas seems to be a cuisine of absent ingredients, but it was varied enough, and good, too, even if endless processions of suckling pig and roast stag and pickled beets can weary even the heartiest appetite. For centuries, well-fed people in Europe made do without a battery of foods we rely on today, and they developed a culinary tradition that survives in most particulars in the

American kitchen: roast meats, boiled vegetables, sturdy breads of all kinds. (Fortunately, other highlights of the early European table, such as the late-Roman delicacy of parboiled flamingo in rotted-fish sauce, are not much replicated today.) Still, when Columbus returned from his first voyage with a ship's hold full of strange new delicacies from the Indies, among them assorted chiles, avocados, tomatoes, maize, mangos, and guavas, he began to fill in gaps in the larder that his contemporaries had not realized they were suffering.

. In the Caribbean, Columbus encountered maize, turkey, peppers, tomatoes, cassava, peanuts, avocado, and guava. He took some of these foods back with him to Spain and then returned—and returned again, carrying goods from one continent to another, altering history with each voyage. A generation after Columbus's arrival in what was with justification called the New World, Hernán Cortés landed on the coast of Mexico with some five hundred soldiers and began his famous—or infamous—strategy of conquering indigenous nations by exploiting old enmities and pitting neighboring and rivalrous peoples against them. Sinking his small fleet in the harbor of Veracruz to let his troops know that there was no turning back, Cortés worked his way inland, one village after another falling before him. In November 1519, having burned a portion of the great city of Cholula, Cortés and his army arrived at the outskirts of Tenochtitlan, the capital of the Aztec empire, a place ringed by irrigation canals and milpas, or fields in which maize and vegetables grew in luxuriant abundance. Cortés wrote admiringly to the king of Spain that the vast city "is much larger than Granada and much stronger, having very good buildings . . . it is much better supplied with provisions such as bread, birds, game, river fish, and vegetables."

Montezuma, the emperor, received Cortés, offering him a meal such as the one Bernardino de Sahagún described in 1530, one that included a dish that Cortés recorded as a taco. In the Spanish of Cortés's time, one meaning of *taco* was "dowel," a piece of turned wood used to join boards and plug a drilled hole. Cortés could have been thinking metaphorically: a taco will fill a hole in your stomach as a dowel fills a hole in a plank. *Taco* may have meant that the food was dowel-shaped—a rolled taco, in other words, of a kind that is popular today in some, but not all, parts of the Southwest. But likelier, Cortés could have been making an effort to pronounce some indigenous word that he'd heard for the dish—in Mixtec, *tlacoyo* referred to a kind of tamale, and Cortés could have been mixing up the words he heard as he was

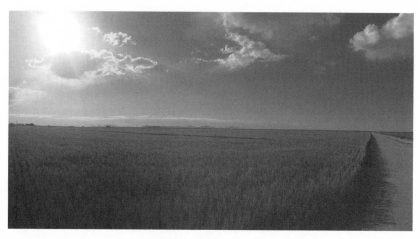

Akimel O'odham (Pima) grain field in south-central Arizona.

introduced to new foods by his hosts. Tlacoyos, a favorite dish in the Mexico City area even today, are masa patties filled with refried beans that look something like small, deflated footballs. These are cooked on a griddle called a comal or on a grill over open flames then garnished with nopalitos, or cooked prickly pear pads, and salsa, all things that would have been familiar to Montezuma but still exotic to the Spanish newcomers.

A taco, as we know it, is obviously a variation on the theme of the tlacoyo, which in turn is a variation on the theme of the tamale. But whether Cortés actually had a taco as we know it remains a subject of historical mystery, for it would have been something akin to serving a visiting head of state to the White House a can of pork and beans, something known by an altogether less neutral name by soldiers in the field. The historian Ross Hassig has speculated that tortillas, the basis of the taco, evolved at least in part out of military necessity: Armies on the march, as we saw as recently as the Civil War in this nation, need to forage constantly in order to keep themselves fed, so any army capable of carrying provisions and still moving swiftly enjoys a tactical advantage. In the case of the tortilla, easily folded and stored in a kit bag, a protein-rich ration allowed Aztec armies to range widely and conquer distant cities, extending their empire to the Pacific Coast, up the Gulf Coast, and south to the Isthmus of Tehuantepec, with vassal and client states radiating Aztec influence far away from Tenochtitlan.

Tlacoyos

The tlacoyo is an ancestral form of the taco, one of those near-universal dishes in which a grain coating surrounds a filling of some sort. In this case, the filling is based on black beans, but, as with the taco, countless variations are possible.

REFRIED BEANS
2 cups dry black beans, picked over and rinsed
2 small white onions, diced
2 teaspoons salt
⅓ cup olive oil or lard

Bring beans, half the onions, and salt to a boil in 4 cups water. Lower heat and simmer for two hours. Drain and allow beans to cool, then purée in a blender. Heat oil in a skillet and cook the rest of the onions until translucent, then add the puréed beans. Simmer for 15–20 minutes, stirring occasionally.

SALSA
8 roasted tomatoes
½ cup diced white onion
3 serrano or jalapeño peppers
1 cup epazote or spinach leaves, loosely packed

Cortés, of course, repaid Montezuma's hospitality badly. He and his men feasted on pineapple, vanilla, peppers, squash, gourds, chia, corn, beans, and tomatoes at the emperor's table, as well as more unusual foods such as salamander larvae and algae from Lake Texcoco. They drank pulque, or fermented agave juice, and were among the first Europeans to smoke tobacco. They even ate food soaked in human blood, Cortés noted, although it moved some of his men to retch.

Cortés then imprisoned and then killed his host. Cortés did so soberly and thoughtfully, for, as his contemporary López de Gomara recorded, the "stoutly built" conquistador "was very fond of eating, but temperate in his drinking."

Cortés, whom López de Gomara added could endure hunger without complaint when he had to, then oversaw the conquest of Mexico and the

½ cup olive oil
1 ½ teaspoon salt

Place vegetables in a blender and purée until smooth. Heat oil in a skillet, then cook the puréed vegetables, simmering on low heat for about 15 minutes.

TLACOYOS
1 pound masa for tortillas
½ cup refried beans
1 tablespoon corn or vegetable oil
8 squash blossoms
1 avocado, cubed
2 tablespoons queso fresco or queso blanco

Divide masa into eight equal portions. Roll into balls, then flatten each masa ball into a patty the size of a small corn tortilla. Place 1 tablespoon refried beans in the center and roll the patty into a cylinder. Press each cylinder into an oval shape, about ¼ inch thick.

In a heavy-bottomed skillet, heat oil, then cook the tlacoyos over low heat for about 4–5 minutes on a side. Spoon squash blossoms, salsa, avocado, and queso over the cooked tlacoyos.

Adapted from Hugo Ortega, *Street Food of Mexico* (Bright Sky Press, 2012)

Christianization of Montezuma's former subjects. In 1528, caught up in court intrigues and legal tangles, he briefly returned to Spain, taking that mysterious Aztec spice called chocolatl with him, the product of a tree that Cortés called *cacap*, "which bears a fruit somewhat like almonds." Not liking its bitterness, members of the Spanish court added sugar to this chocolate, as they called it, and another great worldwide addiction was born.

From the indigenous American point of view, the change was transformative, too. Columbus had brought wheat bread with him on his first voyage. On his second, he brought wheat. On that and subsequent voyages in the first decades of their presence in the Americas, Europeans brought all sorts of food crops and livestock species, from radishes and chickpeas to chickens and goats.

In some instances, they would be disappointed. With the exception of the coastal plane of Sonora and the high plateaus around Mexico City, for instance, most of Spanish North America was not well suited to growing wheat. That limited access to the crop, but not its popularity. The same was true of olives, which also had difficulty finding a congenial home until the Spanish settled in California two centuries after Cortés's conquest of the Valley of Mexico.

In those early years, the Spanish brought horses, cows, sheep, goats, rabbits, chickens, pigs, dogs, and cats. In Mexico and later in the southwest, they found an ideal climate for livestock production, particularly sheep, with huge flocks raised along the great valleys north of Mexico City radiating into what is now the United States. Churro and merino sheep from there were of legendary quality, and their descendants formed the basis of a livestock industry that would flourish in the region up to and including the time that Americans would introduce angora and other varieties into the mix.

They brought sugarcane, a native of Indonesia that was grown in North Africa in antiquity and introduced to Spain by its Moorish conquerors. It did not grow particularly well there, but it certainly did in the Spanish colonies of the Canary Islands, whence it was introduced by Christopher Columbus into the New World. It did not take long before Spanish plantations were established throughout the Caribbean Islands and the coast of Mexico, and sugarcane production became a powerful stimulus for the growth of the slave industry in Spanish America. Sugar, historians have observed, is the first colonial crop, establishing a template that other crops such as rice, tobacco, and cotton would follow: production on large plantations using monoculture and forced labor, translating the Spanish feudal system to a new continent.

In time, the sugar industry would reach the fringes of the Southwest, for sugarcane grew well on the coast of Texas, but even there its cultivation was not widespread, and most sugar was imported into the Southwest, then as now. Sugar was especially well suited to places where other European crops did not grow well, such as olives and wheat, which the Spanish tried to grow in Cuba and the coasts of Central America without success. Hernán Cortés had vast coastal plantations in Mexico, for instance, on which he tried to grow grapes. They did not do particularly well in that humid area, and, in any event, the king of Spain gave in to demands from Spanish wine merchants, outlawing the production of wine in the New World. This was a means of protecting growers back home, and for the first century of Spanish rule in the New World, the conquistadors and their descendants were drinking Spanish wine and not homegrown stuff.

Other plants and crops arrived gradually. Basil, grown for millennia in the Mediterranean, was planted in Spanish household gardens everywhere such gardens existed. There is magic to basil, and in Mexico it is traditionally planted in dooryards to ward off any evil that happens to be abroad. Basil is now reckoned to be the fifth most commonly used medicinal plant in Mexico today, used to combat earache and other pains, as well as to ward off less tangible woes—and, incidentally, to discourage mosquitoes from sticking around, for the phenols in basil are displeasing to those noxious mosquitoes. Also capable of chasing away illness, as the old saying has it, were apples, cultivated for thousands of years in Central Asia and spread commercially along the Silk Route into Europe.

Europeans were carving pathways not only into North America but also into Asia and Africa. With that exploration came many new food crops. From Africa, for example, came coffee, which was native to the area around the Horn of Africa. It had been cultivated in Yemen and other ports on the Indian Ocean for a couple hundred years before the Europeans encountered it, its Arabic name, *qahwah*, being a word for wine—wine, of course, being religiously taboo but widely enjoyed all the same. Once discovered, coffee became a crop in much demand, and its cultivation spread into the Americas. In the same way, rice, native to East Asia, was grown in the Po valley of northern Italy soon after its introduction from China. It, too, was brought to the Americas and grown in small quantities along the coasts, eventually becoming a minor staple of agriculture in coastal Texas and California.

Among the most important of all the foods introduced into the New World were Old World animals, especially cattle. Criollo cattle came to the New World with Columbus on his second voyage, and they proved immensely adaptable to local conditions, especially to the arid conditions in the interior of Mexico and the Southwest; today cattle breeders are wedding the descendants of those criollos to other breeds to prepare them for a changing, warming climate. Following their introduction, great herds of cattle proliferated in the Spanish colonies, introducing much-prized sources of animal protein and quickly transforming the diet of the indigenous peoples. In Mexico,

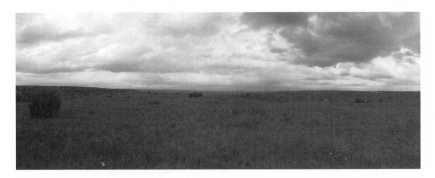

The vast grasslands of Texas and other parts of the Southwest were immediately hospitable to Spanish livestock herds.

cattle ranches tended to concentrate in the valleys between mountainous mining settlements, which provided a ready market for beef and other meats. As the Spanish pressed north into what is now the Southwest, they borrowed the African technique—for so many of the techniques and even words of ranching are ultimately of African origin—of allowing cattle to range freely in the wide-open, unfenced country that, while technically owned by the crown, was really the province of wealthy private individuals. There the cattle browsed on wild vegetation, living more or less unhindered until driven to the slaughterhouse. The ranches thus established were vast, inspiring their descendant ranches in Texas; one ranch in the borderland Mexican state of Coahuila was fourteen million acres in extent. So plentiful were cattle on that northern frontier that they were often slaughtered simply for their hides alone, their meat left for the coyotes and turkey vultures.

An ancillary food derived from those millions of head of Old World livestock was cheese. By definition, all mammals give milk, but not all animal milk has been used to make cheese, and many peoples around the world have chosen not to include cheese in their diets. That wasn't so of the inhabitants of the ancient Sahara, though, where the first archaeological evidence of cheesemaking comes from, dating back more than seven thousand years ago with milk provided courtesy of goats, the first animals to be domesticated in the North African desert. By the time the pyramids were built, cheesemaking had become important to the Egyptian agricultural economy, and cheese has been found tucked into the wrappings of four-thousand-year-old mummies, apparently as a snack for the afterlife. From Africa, cheesemaking traveled far and wide into Europe and western Asia, and the Spanish introduced it to Mexico, and later the Southwest, from very nearly the moment they arrived.

A cheese found in every Mexican restaurant and market today is queso blanco, or white cheese, a variety of which is called queso Chihuahua, or Chihuahua cheese, so named for the Mexican state in which ranching is most preeminent. It is not only delicious but also miraculous, to trust the Southwestern folklorist Jim Griffith. One day a cowboy, a vaquero, in Chihuahua was out riding fences one day when lightning blew a leg off his horse. The horse keeled over. The cowboy rummaged around in his saddlebag and produced a slab of white cheese, holding it above his head and waiting for the next stroke of lightning, which immediately followed—because lightning, of course, always strikes twice in the same place. The lightning melted the cheese, which the cowboy applied to the horse's leg, gluing it back onto its body, and off the two rode, none the worse for the experience.

What pushed the Spanish and Portuguese, and then the other European powers, out into the world? One answer lies in climate, and in a story that will take a little time in the telling. At the dawn of the last millennium, a European wine connoisseur would have sought fine vintages, as today, in Italy, Germany, and France—but also in southern England, then a land dotted with flourishing vineyards. Heat-loving beech trees carpeted Europe far into Scandinavia; Viking ships crossed an iceberg-free ocean to ice-free harbors in Greenland and Newfoundland; farmers enjoyed twice-annual harvests of wheat and other grains; and chroniclers recorded a succession of long, glorious summers and mild winters.

All that changed in the mid-twelfth century, when a cooling trend set in over the Northern Hemisphere. The trend reduced the average annual temperature by only a few degrees, but that was enough to change the face of three continents. Over the next three centuries, England lost its storied vineyards to the cold. In central China, orange groves and mulberry trees froze, chilling a citrus- and silk-based economy that had endured for generations. Glaciers in the Alps, the Himalayas, the Rockies grew by yards, then miles, in just a few years. The Vikings abandoned their colonies in Greenland and North America when the ground became too hard even to bury the dead.

Tamales

I first heard this joke at a friend's house in the barrio of South Tucson, then saw it spread to become a holiday meme in the Christmas season of 2014: "A dozen friends are coming over. I'd better make 50,000 tamales." This recipe from my friend's kitchen yields just a couple of tamales per visitor, but it can be adjusted easily.

1 ½ to 2 pounds beef brisket or roast
1 small jar pitted green olives
2 tablespoons canola or olive oil
1 medium yellow onion, diced
2 Yukon gold potatoes, diced and then parboiled
1 teaspoon dried oregano
1 teaspoon cumin powder
1 teaspoon red chile powder
1 ½ cups hot water
24 dried corn husks
Prepared masa dough for two dozen tamales
Grated Monterey jack, pepper jack, or Chihuahua cheese (queso blanco)

Brown beef in canola oil in a skillet or dutch oven. Transfer to the oven or a crockpot and cook in water until the beef is stringy and falls apart with a fork. Add spices, onion, potato, and olives and cook for another hour or so.

Take a corn husk, pointed side toward you, and spread about ¼ cup masa across it with a spoon, leaving a border of husk on all sides. Put a generous spoonful of the meat mixture in the middle of the husk. Fold the corn husk toward the center until the meat mixture is wrapped in dough. Tie the folded tamale with kitchen string. Place on a rack over a cookie sheet filled with water and steam in the oven for an hour or so, then allow to cool for 15 minutes. Serve warm.

The effects were disastrous. In a time of reduced crop yields, prices of grain shot up, and for the first time in generations Europe knew famine and malnutrition. What little grain that could be stored developed a cold-tolerant blight called ergot, which, among other effects, produced symptoms of madness—symptoms that were often interpreted as proof of demonic possession. With the gnawing pain of hunger came widespread social unrest, and peasant rebellions and small-scale wars became the norm. At the same time, those powers that could afford the expense mounted expeditions to far-off continents, seeking to establish colonies in warmer climes. Even then, Columbus and the explorers who followed him found, even in the Caribbean, cold waters and depleted shoals and forests wherever they went.

Better times came in the late fifteenth century and the arrival of warmer weather, a time that, not coincidentally, brought the period of economic and cultural expansion we now call the High Renaissance. It was just at that time that the awareness of the New World exploded into the Old and just at that time that the goods of the New World and markets for its more durable exports—gold, especially, and silver—found a vast consumer audience in the European homeland.

This meant that there was wealth, and plenty of it, to be had in the New World. Some sought it in mining, the source of much global fortune for centuries following the landing of the conquistadors. Some sought it in agriculture, as with those coastal plantations of Cortés's. And some found it in entrepreneurialism, such as the forward-thinking oceanfarers who established the galleon trade between Acapulco and Manila in the late sixteenth century, one that would thrive as goods were exchanged between Spain's North American colonies and Asia until shortly before Mexico achieved independence nearly three centuries later.

That happy time was interrupted, back in Europe, in a spasm of religious intolerance, witch-hunting, and warfare, all accompanied by a return of the cold—and, indeed, the arrival of temperatures such as Europe had not seen since the age of the Neanderthals. The Dutch painter Pieter Breughel the Elder recorded the onset of that fierce cold snap with his paintings of frozen rivers and swirling armies of half-starved, half-mad villagers, and he was not exaggerating by much: With the advent of the renewed "Little Ice Age," as later scholars would come to call it, came extreme storms, drought, the return of famine and civil war, and the desperate search for someone to blame. So it was that thousands of Europeans were put to death as witches in the cold decades between 1550 and 1620, a hysteria that extended to the British colonies of New England.

Volcanoes, shifts in ocean currents and temperatures, unanticipated climatic heating and cooling all had their effects on world history during the time that Europe was busily conquering the Americas. The Little Ice Age ended as quickly as it arrived, turning from a time of cold to one of temperate weather and increased fertility in only a decade, lessening Europe's need for American foodstuffs but producing a time of prosperity that saw plenty of room for luxury items such as tobacco and chocolate. In an age of rapid global climate change today, we can only hope that traumatic shifts will be followed by similarly good times to come.

Columbus sailed with men whose family names are common in the Southwest today: García, Ortíz, Pérez, Romero, Bernal, Martínez, Fernández, Mendoza. Throughout the sixteenth century, their descendants prospered and multiplied, intermarrying with Native peoples and spreading outward from the Gulf Coast and the Valley of Mexico. By the end of the century, they were poised to move still farther northward, and so it was that on April 30, 1598, a nobleman named Don Juan de Oñate, the son of a wealthy mine owner from Zacatecas, lay claim to the lands north of the Río Grande in the name of King Philip II of Spain. Crossing the river at what is now El Paso, Texas, Oñate and an expedition of more than four hundred soldiers and their families—his own household including a wife who was descended from both Montezuma and Cortés—moved north, driving several thousand head of criollo cattle, pigs, sheep, and other livestock along with them. At points they followed the path of a conquistador named Francisco de Coronado, who half a century earlier had gone off in quest of the golden cities that Cabeza de Vaca had promised and who had been broken physically and mentally for his troubles.

Oñate had gold in mind as well, but he also intended to bring the wild north country under the subjugation of the cross and the Spanish crown. It was a difficult and hungry passage to the north, so much so that Oñate was moved to name one indigenous village along the river Socorro, or "succor," because the people there had an abundance of corn that they shared with the Spanish. Eventually the expedition arrived in the pleasingly fertile river valley above what is now Albuquerque, country that reminded those few of his number who had seen the old country of Andalusia, and moved in among Pueblo Indian farms among which grazed churro sheep that had been left behind as Coronado's men pressed northeastward out onto the Great Plains.

Like Cortés, Oñate was soon enough swept up in political intrigue, and in 1607 he was forced to travel to Spain to stand tall before a bureaucratic inquest. His successor, Pedro de Peralta, founded a new city near those farm fields, and in 1609 Santa Fe became the capital of the new territory of New Mexico. The Spanish there introduced European methods of crop production, bringing a different kind of order to the ancient agriculture of the upper Rio Grande. They also introduced Moorish systems of irrigation control, combining the technologies of North Africa and the Roman Empire to develop a system of irrigated agriculture that is still prevalent in New Mexico today.

Not that the Native peoples of the Southwest were strangers to irrigation: Both the Hohokam of southern Arizona and the Pueblo peoples along the great river had developed hydraulic civilizations of a staggering complexity that, as the historian Karl Wittfogel observed, had to have entailed not just great engineering skills but also a hierarchical social organization to keep the ditches cleared, the water flowing, and the produce fanning out to distant markets. Still, that productive river valley became even more productive with those Moorish/Roman *acequias*, so much so that an inspector for the Spanish crown, a prelate named Alonso de Benavides, was moved to report of the country around Santa Fe: "All this land is most fertile, yielding with very great abundance all that is planted in it—corn, wheat, beans, lentils, garbanzos, broad beans, vetches, squashes, watermelons, cantaloupes, cucumbers, all sorts of garden stuff, cabbages, lettuce, carrots, artichokes, garlic, onions, prickly pears, hedgehog cacti, plums, apricots, peaches, nuts, acorns, mulberries, and many others which I won't mention to avoid tediousness."

Tedious or not, it is worth noting that the rich blend of crops that Benavides enumerated was made up of foods from the Old World (cantaloupes and garlic) and the New (corn and prickly pears). That pattern would continue as the upper Rio Grande began to fill with Spanish farms and estates and then elsewhere in the Southwest over the next two centuries as missions and other settlements were established. One of the greatest champions of this effort to bring the northern borderlands of New Spain under proper Spanish rule was a Jesuit named Eusebio Francisco Kino, who came to the territory known as the Pimería Alta, what is now southern Arizona, in 1687.

A German-speaking Italian from the Tyrol, Kino was renowned as an ascetic, intellectual soldier of Christ who used neither salt nor spices, wore sackcloth, and slept on a horse blanket. The emphasis might have fallen on "soldier," for Kino was also renowned for his toughness and military shrewdness, and in the thousands on thousands of miles that he logged on what was called the Rim of Christendom on foot and horseback, he was never known to complain.

Kino's chief interest was in establishing missions, a combination of church, ranch, and fortress, from northern Sonora to the Gila River, in the vicinity of present-day metropolitan Phoenix. These missions were a day's ride apart, radiating northward in a system that commenced in Mexico City and eventually extended all the way to San Francisco to the west and San Antonio to the east. The missions were meant to be self-sufficient and to feed a population of missionaries, Indians, Spanish settlers, and soldiers. Still, they needed to be supplied, and for many years any missionary traveling into New Mexico from what is now Mexico proper was under orders to bring ten heifers, ten sheep, and forty-eight chickens, with any room left in their wagons after packing them with grain and other essentials used, ideally, to stow away a few pounds of sugar, chocolate, and other luxury goods. To the south, in turn, were sent surplus wheat and corn, cotton and wool, piñon nuts from the New Mexico high country, hides from the abundant pronghorn, elk, and bison herds, and finally slaves, often children captured in raids against supposedly hostile Indian villages.

Kino established a policy that other missions would follow, called *reducción*, or "reduction," by which Indian villages were relocated to the missions and the people transformed, effectively, into Spanish farmers. The policy was not always welcomed, particularly because in many instances the indigenous farmers were discouraged from growing food plants that were culturally important to them and instead put to work growing barley and other, to them, exotic crops—and more, to raising livestock, which brought the benefit of new animal proteins but also occasioned the destruction of traditional ways of life. From time to time, the Indians rebelled; they did so in 1680 in New Mexico, when the Pueblo Revolt put an end to Spanish rule along the Rio Grande for a dozen years, and again in Sonora in 1751, when an O'odham uprising briefly threatened to drive the Spanish from the region. It is small wonder that when Indian rebellions occurred, a chief feature was the mass slaughter of mission livestock.

Sometimes cattle became a problem in their abundance. Wrote Pedro Lorenzo de Cárdenas, a colonial priest in Matapé, Sonora, forty years before Kino arrived,

The constant presence of the cattle around Banachari produced concern and alarm among the owners and managers of the cattle because of the damage that they were doing [to the crops] in spite of the care the dark-skinned cowboys exercised while they were driving the cattle up towards the high mountains that look out onto [the Río] Sonora, and in spite of the vigilance of the Indians who were guarding the wheat and their own cornfields. The Indians finally became weary of planting only to have the livestock eat their crops and the priest grew exasperated and irritated trying to settle arguments. Disgusted, the Indians ceased planting at the said site of Banachari.

Horses, too, were overly abundant on the northern edges of New Spain. A missionary named Juan Morfí found *mesteño*, or feral—the word gives us our *mustang*—horses beyond counting within sight of the mission at El Paso, so many that, from a horse's point of view, it was "the most populous country in the world." The horses had overgrazed the range all along the river, he added, and nonnative plants such as stonecrop and filaree were moving in to fill the empty spaces in the landscape. Spanish livestock proved an attractive nuisance in other ways, encouraging raids of Indians outside the mission system. Apaches and Comanches traveled down from far to the north precisely because those herds of fat cattle and horses proved to be theirs for the taking, and this in turn, as ethnohistorian Thomas Sheridan observes, "created an ever more militarized frontier, one that Spain could never quite control."

More soldiers meant, naturally, the increased possibility of hostilities with not just Apaches and Comanches but also the "reduced" peoples under Spanish control. Good missions, such as those administered by Father Kino, were frictionless, but bad ones, including, notoriously, missions under the command of the recently canonized Junípero Serra, were full of conflict, their resident farmers little more than slaves. Wrote a condescending French visitor to the mission at Monterey, California, in 1786,

At noon the dinner was announced by the bell; the Indians quitted their work, and sent to fetch their rations in the same vessels as at breakfast; but this second mess was thicker than the first; there was mixed in it corn and maize, and peas and beans; the Indians name it *poussole* [i.e., *posole*]. They return again to their labor from two o'clock till four or five; afterwards they attend evening prayers, which continue near an hour, and is followed by a new ration of *atole* like that at breakfast. These three distributions are sufficient for the subsistence of the far greater number of Indians, and this very economical soup might perhaps be very profitably adopted in our years of scarcity; some seasoning would certainly be necessary to be added to it, their whole knowledge of cookery consisting in being able to roast the grain before it is reduced into meal. As the Indian women have no vessels of earth or metal for this operation, they perform it in large baskets made of bark, over a little lighted charcoal; they turn these vessels with so much rapidity and address, that they effect the swelling and bursting of the grain without burning the basket, though it is made of very combustible materials: and we can testify, that the best roasted coffee does not nearly equal the exactness with which these women prepare their corn. It is distributed to them every morning, and the smallest dishonesty when they give it out is punished by whipping.

Most newcomers to other parts of the Spanish Southwest, however, found it a happier place than all that, its people welcoming everywhere. Even in California, where it would be so often met with the bad faith of Cortés, the hospitality of the indigenous peoples was noteworthy. Wrote Juan Crespi, on arriving at the site of the mission that would lie at the heart of what is now Los Angeles,

> We pitched camp on the left bank of the river. On its right bank there is a populous village of Indians, who received us with great friendliness. Fifty-two of them came to the camp, and their chief told us by signs which we understood very well that we must come to live with them; that they would make houses for us, and provide us with food such as antelope, hares, and seeds. . . . The chief gave us two baskets of seeds, already made into *pinole*, together with a string of beads made of shells such as they wear. I called this place the sweet name of Jesus de los Temblores, because we experienced here a horrifying earthquake, which was repeated four times during the day.

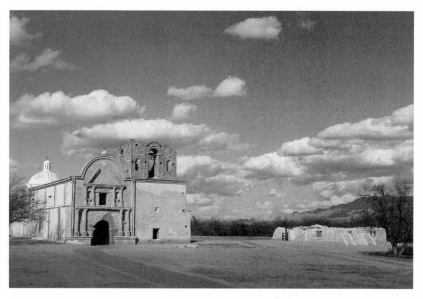

Tumacacori Mission, a Spanish outpost along Arizona's Santa Cruz River, established in 1691.

Earthquakes notwithstanding, the lands were astonishingly fertile, too, even in the deepest of the deserts, given water and the time necessary to adjust the soil for Spanish crops and trees. Eusebio Francisco Kino and other missionaries planted apples, pears, walnuts, medlars, hazelnuts, figs, grapes, chestnuts, plums, peaches, pistachios, almonds, cherries, quinces, oranges bitter and sweet, and many other plants known within the confines of the Roman world and spread throughout the empire wherever they could grow. Apricots, brought to Europe from the Middle East during the Crusades, were another favorite of the missionaries, adding to the more ordinary food crops. Kino was pleased to note the spread of watermelons and muskmelons, Old World plants, throughout the Pimería. They proved an instant hit among the O'odham, who could grow them out in the desert in traditional floodwater fields and store them throughout the year. Kino even brought chile peppers into his missions, for although the ancient ancestors of the O'odham would have known chiles, they seem to have made less use of them than their Puebloan neighbors to the east, who were avid for the heat.

New Mexico Apple Pie

Since the 1920s, the hamlet of Pie Town, New Mexico, has been a haven for lovers of the signature dish evoked in its very name. Today a couple of well-appointed diners continue the tradition, serving up delicious pies. This recipe comes from one of them, the Pie Town Café, featuring a fine blend of Mesoamerican chiles and the Central Asian apples brought into the region by the Spanish.

FOR A 9-INCH PIE:
6 cups peeled sliced apples (preferably a mix of Granny Smiths and
  Fuji or Galas)
½ cup of flour
½ cup of turbinado sugar
2 tablespoons cinnamon
½ teaspoon dried ground ginger
½ teaspoon fresh ground nutmeg
2 ounces fresh lemon juice
2 ounces hot green chili
2 ounces piñon nuts
Egg wash: 1 egg and 2 ounces water
2 tablespoons turbinado sugar

Mix all ingredients well in a bowl and let them sit for 20 minutes to meld. Fill the bottom crust and cover with a full top crust. Poke the top crust with a fork to vent. Brush with egg wash, sprinkle the top with turbinado sugar, and bake in a 375-degree oven for 1 to 1 ½ hours, turning the pie every 20 minutes to get an even golden brown. Look for thick bubbles of juices from the vent holes.

The proprietor adds, "I suggest a scoop of vanilla ice cream or whipped cream. Share with good people and enjoy!"

The Columbian exchange was not a seamless process. When the Tongva people met Crespi in what is now Los Angeles, they gave him welcoming gifts. When Crespi returned the kindness, they kept the trade goods he offered, but they secretly buried the foreign food he gave them. "It was not that the natives feared deliberate poisoning," wrote the eminent California anthropologist A. L. Kroeber, "but they were evidently imbued with a strong conviction similar to that of the Mohave, who believed that every nation had its own peculiar food and that for one to partake of the characteristic nourishment of the other or to mingle with its women, or in fact associate in any prolonged contact, was bound in the very nature of things to bring sickness."

Contact induced sicknesses of many sorts. Still, a well-maintained mission proved a cornucopia. Wrote one Spanish military officer in 1731, "In the places where water is sufficient and the soil suitable for their respective cultivations, the following have prevailed: the olive, lemon, orange, peach, pomegranate, fig, apple, guava, yellow sapota, watermelon, muskmelon, pumpkin (also squash), date palms, wheat, corn, rice, and various kinds of vegetables." In other words, in many parts of what is now the Southwest, people were eating better than they were in Europe—a fact that would soon send many more Europeans into the region.

4. **La Frontera**

Within a few years of Christopher Columbus's arrival in the West Indies, Native American words were entering European languages: from Taino, *mahís*; from Arawakan, *tabaco*; from Quechan, *papa*; from Nahuatl, *kakáwa*, *tomatl*, and *chocolatl*. Turkeys graced European barnyards, even if the bird was believed to come from India or Guinea, and corn was soon flourishing in plots along the Guadalquivir and Po.

Within a few decades of Columbus's arrival, Europeans were on the frontier of what is now the Southwest—and not long after that, were settling in the region. They and those who followed them brought the manifold fruits of the Columbian exchange into a part of the world that had already seen an advanced agricultural tradition many millennia old. They made farms and gardens that observed no distinctions between foods because of their national or continental origins. The Jesuit missionary and explorer Eusebio Francisco Kino alone introduced barley, wheat, cabbage, lettuce, carrots, garlic, leeks, onions, turnips, black-eyed peas, garbanzos, lentils, radishes, apples, apricots, oranges, peaches, plums, pomegranates, watermelons, mustard, mint, coriander, walnuts, and sugarcane into the gardens of the northern frontier. Many of these had been introduced to the New World in turn by Christopher Columbus himself, brought over on his second voyage in

1493. They were growing abundantly and vigorously a century and a half after Kino's time, when an American surveyor passing through Tucson in 1852, John Bartlett, recorded gardens full of wheat, corn, peas, beans, lentils, apples, pears, peaches, grapes, onions, and pumpkins, commenting that in "such a fertile valley" all these things would of course grow well. All that was needed was a little more clemency of climate—a truism that had a sardonic reply in the Southwestern saw, "Yes, but all hell needs is water."

A characteristic quality of Southwestern cuisine is that it is simple—but deceptively so, since it involves a body of learning and experience that dates back thousands of years. Consider that complex simplicity as it plays out, for instance, in a memory of tortillas by El Paso writer José Antonio Burciaga:

> In the mercado where my mother shopped, we frequently bought *taquitos de nopalitos*, small tacos filled with diced cactus, onions, tomatoes, and jalapeños. Our friend Don Toribio showed us how to make delicious, crunchy taquitos with dried, salted pumpkin seeds. When you had no money for the filling, a poor man's taco could be made by placing a warm tortilla on the left palm, applying a sprinkle of salt, then rolling the tortilla up quickly with the fingertips of the right hand. My own kids put peanut butter and jelly on tortillas, which I think is truly bicultural. And speaking of fast foods for kids, nothing beats a quesadilla, a tortilla grilled-cheese sandwich.

Simplicity and poverty combined to produce, in Mexico, the distinct belief that Mexican cuisine was somehow below the culinary standards of more desirable Continental cuisine, especially French. Until the 1950s and a revival of nationalism, Mexican dishes often appeared tucked in the back of Mexican cookbooks, in the section headed "*indígenista.*" The arrival of Josefina Vélazquez de León's cookbook *Platillos regionales de la República Mexicana* in 1946 signaled the beginning of that change, and it made room for dishes from the northern borderlands, which sometimes took different forms from their counterparts farther north across the international line.

That simplicity, as much as anything else, has allowed Southwestern cuisine to hop from kitchen to kitchen and continent to continent. There are distinct food regions in the Southwest, to be sure, as we will see. Still, the

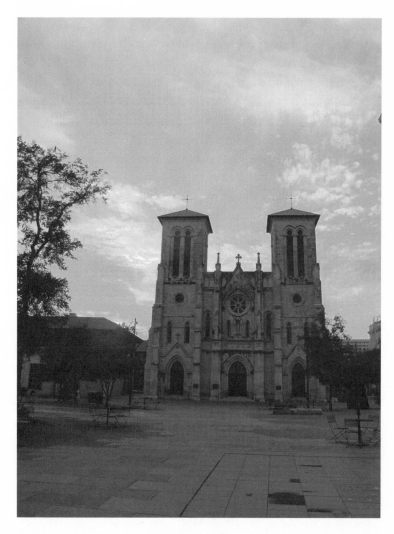

Cathedral of San Fernando, San Antonio, Texas. Construction of the colonial church began in 1738.

hottest and, truth be told, one of the most memorable salsas I ever ate was in the main train station in Zurich, Switzerland, where a young woman, Swiss German on her father's side, served up a wonderful blend of peppers, tomatoes, onions, and cilantro that her Mexican mother had prepared in her kitchen. It was a perfect remedy for that cold, rainy alpine morning—and for homesickness as well.

In 1846, following the close of the war with Mexico, an American newcomer to the Southwest, an eighteen-year-old named Susan Magoffin, described the typical meals that she was served in Santa Fe and points south along the Camino Real. She was a little alarmed when first presented with a stack of tortillas covered in a much-used napkin alongside a large bowl of stewed meat and onions. When no cutlery appeared at the table, she divined that the tortillas were meant to be dipped into the chile, a thought that set off alarms of cultural collision. "My heart sickened, to say nothing of my stomach," she wrote. Matters did not improve when she was brought a dish of green chile: "There were a few mouthfuls taken," she said, "for I could not eat a dish so strong and unaccustomed to my palate."

In no time, though, Susan acclimated to the new diet and the new ways of New Mexico, and she began to enjoy the food she encountered, becoming one of the first known Anglo aficionados of a regional cuisine characterized by smoky, fiery chiles. A typical meal, she wrote, involved beans, peppers, tomatoes, rice, lamb or mutton, pork, chicken, onions, cabbage, corn that usually took the form of tortillas, and wheat that usually took the form of bread of some sort—in short, very much what we think of as being Southwestern cuisine today, involving ingredients from around the world, with the addition that the people she met drank chocolate throughout the day and wine at night. They were also spicing their foods in ways that we think of as being Southwestern today, using Old World and New World ingredients such as chile, onion, basil, cumin, coriander, and oregano, fruits of the Columbian exchange in all their brilliant diversity and abundance.

On feast days, they ate much the same foods, but more of them. On the feast day of Saint Gabriel, for instance, a neighbor brought Susan a bowl of carne de carnero, or mutton, along with some stewed chicken and bread pudding studded with yellow and red grapes. Spanish people on the frontier enjoyed a treat as much as anyone else, but their favorites at first were things that were brought in at considerable expense. For example, rice pudding depended on rice that was grown in the Indies, if not in Asia, while cinnamon was brought in from the Spice Islands by way of routes established by the galleon trade. The milk in that pudding was a luxury, for cow's milk was not often drunk except by human infants on the frontier and even then not often. Cooks soon learned to adapt, however, coming up with wonderful dishes such as cajeta, which is made of scorched goat milk to which a sugary syrup is added, producing a kind of caramel. Susan Magoffin described this as "a dish made of boiled milk and seasoned with cinnamon and nutmeg, and it was very good, the recipe I should like."

Whether the recipe had any vanilla in it, she does not say. The vanilla bean had long before traveled to Europe, carried there by envoys of Hernán Cortés, and been enthusiastically adopted by bakers everywhere after vanilla plantations in Réunion and other colonies helped reduce the price. Vanilla was familiar on the northern frontier of New Spain as well, though expensive. Not until late in the nineteenth century would food scientists develop a means of extracting vanillin from sources other than the orchid-like vanilla plant, setting vanilla on course to being the most common dessert flavoring in the world kitchen.

Green Chile Stew

Erna Fergusson (1888–1964) was an Anglo devotee of all things Southwestern. As a girl, she lived in La Glorieta, the oldest hacienda in Albuquerque. On returning to the city after a time in Washington, DC, she began to write books about the Native Americans and Hispanos of New Mexico, including her *Mexican Cookbook*, first published in 1934. The recipe she offers here for green chile stew is a definitive blend of Southwestern traditions.

1 pound round steak cut in small cubes
1 tablespoon flour
2 tablespoons lard
1 small onion, chopped
4–6 green chiles, chopped
1 clove garlic, chopped fine
2 cups boiling water
1 teaspoon salt
1/8 teaspoon pepper

Sprinkle steak with flour and brown steak and onion in hot lard. Add chiles, garlic, water, and seasoning. Simmer about 30 minutes. If necessary, add more boiling water.

A small can of tomatoes may be added.

The descendants of Oñate and company had long since made homes in the upper Rio Grande Valley, and throughout the Southwest, by the time Susan Magoffin came to the region. They had developed a style of cooking different from that farther south and elsewhere along the borderlands, one that particularly favored pork, from an animal more readily accessible to small farmers than were land-hungry cattle.

New Mexico cuisine today is characterized by meats long stewed in chile, so long, in fact, that they've fallen off the bone, their fats long since rendered in the sauce and their tendons liquefied. A classic New Mexico example is posole, a stew made of hominy, corn kernels that have been soaked in lime water to puff them up. This hominy is added to a stew made of cubed or diced pork, onions, cumin, oregano, and red chile and then cooked for hours, with broth sometimes added in to keep the stew from drying out. Posole is traditionally served only in cold weather, and it is a standard of the New Mexico table at Christmastime. In Navajo country, which begins an hour's drive west of the Rio Grande, those ingredients are the same save for the substitution of mutton or lamb for pork to make a dish found on menus in places like Gallup and Farmington and guaranteed to warm your stomach on a cold night in the high plateau country.

You can have a fine time in New Mexico simply whipping up the basics of a chile colorado or a chile verde. For the former, red chile pods are seeded and their stems removed, then roasted over a flame or on a grill, and then, once it has cooled, pureed with broth. Chile verde, made with green chile in the same way, typically has the added refinement of removing the skin.

Northerners would disagree, of course, but most connoisseurs hold that the best green chile in New Mexico—and therefore in the world—comes from the lower Rio Grande Valley around the towns of Garfield, Derry, and especially, and famously, Hatch. So prized is Hatch green chile that the state of New Mexico has established a certification program for it as restrictive as the moniker *tequila* is for the distillate of blue agaves. On June 17, 2011, the New Mexico Chile Advertising Act went into effect, with one section holding that it is unlawful for a person to knowingly advertise, describe, label, or offer for sale a product as containing New Mexico chile unless the chile peppers or chile peppers in the product were grown in New Mexico. Whether chile fraud is a widespread problem is secondary to the good advertising that comes from it, and the name "Hatch" on a container is as good an imprimatur as a diner could want.

If there is a single taste that defines the essence of the Southwest, to my mind it is green chile, a taste at once fiery and delicate, smoky and sophisticated. If you have green chile from Hatch, then you really need look no further, though the inquiring eater will of course want to do just that, if only for purposes of comparison.

A taco is a taco, coming in many shapes and forms, embracing many fillings. Just so, the food of Mexico varies widely by region, and the food of the Southwestern subregions that those Mexican regions abut varies, too. Baja California, blessed by the waters of the Pacific Ocean and the Gulf of California, is the home of the shrimp taco. Moreover, it gave rise to the related fish taco, said to be a recent culinary invention, as we will soon see, but probably one that dates back into deep prehistory. Zacatecas boasts pork tacos and Durango beef tacos marinated in a sauce that includes both onions and garlic, a violation of all that is sacred in the cooking of Emilia-Romagna but that works very nicely in the mouth all the same. In Chihuahua, mutton tacos give diners pleasure, while in Sonora beef reigns supreme. In Tamaulipas, bordering the south coast of Texas, you'll find fish again, while in neighboring San Luis Potosí you'll find tacos that would make a vegetarian happy, concocted of cheese, potatoes, scrambled eggs, and chiles hot enough to melt you in your shoes.

There are reasons for that variety, just as there are reasons for the curious fact that no bowl of refried beans ever quite tastes the same from town to town or even street to street. Classically, those gifts of the Central American rainforest are brought to the table courtesy of happy helpings of lard, a marriage of Old World and New World, of the Americas and Eurasia—or, better, of Mesoamerica and Mesopotamia. That lard component is not a requirement, and there are plenty of substitutes for it, one being canola oil—*canola* being a shortened form of *Canadian oil*. Even so, there are some connoisseurs who say that refrieds without lard are inauthentic. A friend of mine who has been a vegetarian for all the more than forty years I have known him, a devotee of bean tostadas, bean burritos, and all the other ways a lard-dripping pot of frijoles refritos can be served, always says to me simply, "Shhh," whenever the porcine subject comes up.

Spell chile like the name of the country, and you are describing a class of peppers but also the dishes made from them: the aforementioned chile colorado, for example, that smoky, earthy red chile stew so beloved in New Mexico and southern Arizona, or chile verde, the lighter green chile potion that is often put to work to liven up stewed chicken or turkey. Spell chile with an *i* at the end, though, and you have crossed the border into Texas—never mind the fact that one of the first occurrences of the word so rendered was across the line in New Mexico and on the deathbed of the renowned frontiersman Kit Carson, whose scribe recorded that he said, a moment before passing away in 1868, "Wish I had time for just one more bowl of chili."

When Frank Tolbert wrote his fine book *A Bowl of Red*, celebrating Texas cuisine, he queried former first lady Lady Bird Johnson about her favorite recipe. She obliged, adding in a note this lovely thought: "My feeling about chili is this—along in November, when the first norther strikes and the skies are gray, along about 5 o'clock in the afternoon, I get to thinking how good chili would taste for supper. It always lives up to expectations. In fact, you don't even mind the cold November winds."

In that book, Tolbert calls the chile-laden concoction called son-of-a-bitch stew "Texas' greatest contribution to civilization." Why the name? Well, the heat may have something to do with it; the phrase may have escaped the mouth of a tenderfoot diner, along with a cascade of steam and fire. More likely the name owes to a cowboy's telling said tenderfoot, when asked what mysterious ingredients went into the stew, "I'll be a son-of-a-bitch if I know all that goes into it. Different cooks put in different things, but it's sure good."

Chile is chili is chile, but with a difference. Chili con carne, or chile peppers with meat, is that "bowl of red," a nicely succinct cowboy phrase that describes a classic, nearly canonical recipe: seared beef left to stew in peppers and onions, with cumin and oregano—the sort of thing that might be prepared as easily in a chuckwagon dutch oven as on a comfortable home hearth. That meat component is important: Whereas a New Mexico chile colorado is sometimes made of peppers alone or with just a little meat, a Texas chili is always a meaty thing, excepting the "vegetarian chili" found on menus here and there. But as to vegetables, a chuckwagon ration would also have included a scoop or two of charro beans—boiled pinto or red beans, that is, cooked with bacon. Allow those beans to creep into the bowl of red, and you have a near-theological controversy: Is chili with beans really chili, or even chile?

That's a matter for purists to decide, but suffice it to say that in a proper Texas chili cookoff of the sort that pepper the social calendar of so many towns in the Lone Star State, you'll find beans served as a side dish.

As for other Texan contributions to Southwestern cuisine, let us not turn our thoughts to fajitas—skirt steak cooked on a hot plate or cast-iron skillet in onions and green peppers—but instead to the delightful variation on chilaquiles called migas, or crumbs. The dish by that name served in central Mexico, where it originated, is a light broth with various bits and pieces of pig meat sopped up with shreds of bolillo, or crusty bread. On the way north to the border, that bolillo was transformed into shreds of stale corn tortilla, the pig parts into scrambled eggs. By the time it got to Austin, where migas is a local favorite, the dish had acquired a topping of cheese, though, like the beans in a bowl of red, there is some discussion about the propriety and traditionalness of that added dairy. There's also a division among cooks as to whether jalapeño or serrano chiles are the way to go, serranos being generally hotter. Either way, migas comes highly recommended as a hangover cure.

California has always been a cornucopia, and the people who moved there from southerly places in New Spain celebrated it as such. The mission fathers who established such colonial outposts as San Gabriel, as we have seen, planted gardens as soon as they could, long before their buildings were

---

Migas

(Serves 4)
12 corn tortillas
Vegetable oil
8–10 eggs, beaten
Salt and pepper to taste
1 diced onion
1 diced tomato
2 diced jalapeño or serrano chiles, roasted

Cut the tortillas into rectangular strips and fry in the vegetable oil to near crispness. Drain on paper towels. Cook eggs until they are just beginning to set. Fold in tortillas and mix, then fold in vegetables.

finished. There, under the guidance of European and Mexican clerics, the Tongva people, whom the Spanish called Gabrieleños, planted wheat, grapes, apples, peaches, corn, and oranges and tended large and growing herds of cattle, horses, and sheep. One soldier in the army of Spain, a man named José Maria Verdugo, was given a land grant for his service near the Mission San Gabriel. His Rancho San Rafael, about thirty-six thousand acres in extent, founded in 1784, is the site of the present-day California city of Glendale.

In its time, Verdugo grew huge quantities of vegetables, fruits, grains, and other crops, establishing a pattern that others, such as the Kentuckian newcomer William Wolfskill, would follow into the nineteenth century. The cattle herds that dotted a thousand hills became vast during the Gold Rush era, though their numbers would be lessened considerably by huge drought in 1862 and again later in the decade. Sheep took the place of cattle during that time, and in the 1870s, most of the cattle and other livestock in the region gave way to large crop cultivation. Helen Hunt Jackson, whose highly influential novel *Ramona* (1884) was sympathetic to both Mexicans and Indians of California, offered a highly romanticized but historically important view of ordinary life among that plenty:

> At last supper was ready—a great dish of spiced beef and cabbage in the center of the table; a tureen of thick soup, with forcemeat balls and red peppers in it; two red earthen platters heaped, one with boiled rice and onions, the other with the delicious *frijoles* so dear to all Mexican hearts; cup glass dishes filled with hot stewed pears, or preserved quinces, or grape jelly; plates of frosted cakes of various sorts; and a steaming silver tea kettle, from which went up an aroma of tea such as had never been bought or sold in all California, the Señora's one extravagance and passion.

Guadalupe Vallejo, a nephew of the eminent Mexican aristocrat Mariano Vallejo, had much the same recollection of life before the supremacy of the Americans. He recalled in 1890 of life in San José,

> No one need suppose that the Spanish pioneers of California suffered many hardships or privations, although it was a new country. They came slowly, and were well prepared to become settlers. All that was necessary

for the maintenance and enjoyment of life according to the simple and healthful standards of those days was brought with them. They had seeds, trees, vines, cattle, household goods, and servants, and in a few years their orchards yielded abundantly and their gardens were full of vegetables. Poultry was raised by the Indians, and sold very cheaply; a fat capon cost only twelve and a half cents. Beef and mutton were to be had for the killing, and wild game was very abundant. At many of the missions there were large flocks of tame pigeons. At the Mission San Jose the fathers' doves consumed a *cental* [100 pounds] of wheat daily, besides what they gathered in the village. The doves were of many colors, and they made a beautiful appearance on the red tiles of the church and the tops of the dark garden walls.

Add all that variety to a generous climate, and it is small wonder that a distinct California cuisine grew up around that early version of farm to table, although always with a little heat to it—or so George Simpson, a British traveler to California just before the American takeover, complained, saying of his host's supper offering that it was "merely a counterpart of the breakfast . . . the same stews, the same frijoles, and the same pepper and garlic, with the same dead-and-alive temperature in every morsel."

It stands to reason that California's indigenous cuisine should have included the bounty of the sea. For millennia, one supposes, the coastal peoples grew corn and then ate fish with it, giving rise to what today we call the fish taco. Yet, in a contest whose rewards are nil but whose stakes are high, there has been claim to more recent authorship of the fish taco, with one party tracing its origins to a fish market in Ensenada, not far below the international border in Baja California Norte, and the other to a seaside food shack in San Felipe, on the Gulf of California. In both cases, the flaky white fish was dipped in a light tempura-like batter, fried, and served in corn tortillas with a topping of mayonnaise and shredded cabbage. In the 1970s, a visiting American college student from San Diego, Ralph Rubio, worked out a recipe and, in 1983, opened a small restaurant in the shell of an abandoned hamburger stand in Mission Bay. Other vendors picked up on the idea, and by the time I first had a fish taco in inland Pasadena a year or two later, the concoction was widespread throughout Southern California. The fish taco is now standard on Mexican-themed menus far within the continental interior,

Calabacitas

2 pounds zucchini (about 6–7 medium)
2 tablespoons olive oil
1 chopped onion
1 tablespoon minced garlic
1 teaspoon dried oregano or verbena
1 cup diced green chile, roasted
2 cups corn kernels
Salt and pepper to taste
Chopped cilantro or Italian parsley

Cut the ends from the zucchini. Quarter the zucchini, then chop into half-inch pieces. In olive oil, cook the onion until translucent. Stir in garlic and oregano and cook for another minute, then fold in the zucchini and chile. Cook about five to ten minutes over low heat until the zucchini is soft but not mushy. Add the corn and cook another minute or two. Top with cilantro or parsley and serve warm as an accompaniment to grilled meat or green enchiladas.

while Rubio's original restaurant has grown into a small chain that serves both fried fish and more healthful grilled versions of fish and shellfish.

An enchilada is a tortilla soaked in chile sauce. That much is stated in its very name. Lay two or three such enchiladas flat on a plate, with extra chile and cheese layered in between each of them, top with a fried egg, and you have a New Mexico–style flat enchilada. Thicken the tortilla into a masa cake, something on the order of a Yankee's corn johnnycake, and you have a Sonoran flat enchilada, a basic meal in Mexican American households throughout southern Arizona—and much more common than the rolled enchilada, the iteration most frequently found in restaurants but, as an exotic item from farther south in Mexico, held to be just a little fancier than a simple home-cooked meal calls for. Turn up the end of the masa cake with a pinch of your thumb and forefinger, and you have a chalupa, the rim serving the purpose of keeping beans and vegetables from sliding off.

Arizona's proximity to Sonora means that its characteristic dishes include wheat and beef. That's a simple proposition. But consider the mystery dish called the burrito. The name, meaning "little burro," dates to 1895, and the first recorded instance of the foodstuff—a soft wheat flour tortilla wrapping a couple of spoonfuls of beans and chicken—finds its setting in Zacatecas, in central Mexico, where it suggested to its unknown inventor the beast of burden so abundant in the Mexican countryside. Perhaps a little burro carried a couple of basketsful of the treat up the hills there to hungry miners. Yet today the burrito is not often found by that name south of the line, while it is a staple on the American side, found on every Mexican menu and as often as not ordered with a filling of beef cooked in red chile.

Deep-fry that burrito, and it becomes something different, a crispy torpedo of goodness. In Tucson, where one restaurant in particular claims to have invented it, it is called the chimichanga, so new that when I moved to the city in 1975 it was the subject of heavy-rotation television ads with a beaming man saying, "if you love chimichangas, I mean *really* love chimichangas . . . " and urging viewers to head to his restaurant—which was not its birthplace. But then, the birthplace of the chimichanga, whose name is translated as "thingamabob," is probably not Tucson, either—and certainly not Santa Fe or Albuquerque, from which renegade New Mexicans have occasionally floated claims of invention. Given that in southern Sonora and towns in neighboring northern Sinaloa, Yaqui people have long been eating smaller versions of the concoction that they call chivichanga, a square of tortilla filled with meat and potatoes and often topped with mayonnaise, it would seem likely that the chimichanga came north with Yaqui people when they crossed the border seeking asylum during a period of genocidal persecution on the part of the Mexican government, settling in several small communities in Tucson and one south of Phoenix. Their arrival in the early 1900s coincides with the first known attestation of the "chimichanga" in Tucson, which, if nothing else, can claim to be to hub out of which missionary chimichanga spokes have radiated out into neighboring Southwestern states—and within the last quarter century, the chimichanga has been turning up on menus everywhere.

So have refried beans, which are a bit of a misnomer, since refrieds are not fried and fried again but are instead fried once—preferably but not necessarily in lard—and then mashed into a creamy texture. A century ago, a young Arizona *tamalera* named Rosaura Castro was so well known for the beans that accompanied her wares that she was able to build a small, local company selling them to Phoenix-area restaurants. In 1961 she sold her company, Rosarita, to a conglomerate but continued to make refried beans by the huge vatful until retiring years later, sending a particular version of that staple food out into kitchens across the Southwest and beyond. Other brands exist, but Rosaritas continue to be the choice of cognoscenti in too much of a hurry to whip up a potful of frijoles themselves.

Common in home kitchens in Arizona, but not often found on restaurant menus, is verdolaga. It is far from a stranger outside of those homes, to be sure: George Washington grew it, and so did Thomas Jefferson, and so did many colonial gardeners in the America of old, from New England to Georgia. So do many modern ones, although, in the United States, usually as an ornamental, in which form you'll find it in garden catalogs as portulaca in several species. Older gardeners would have called one of those species, *Portulaca oleracea*, porcellane, or purslane. In the Deep South, they might even have called it pigweed, as distinct from the amaranth that Southwestern Anglo farmers called by the same name. And they would have grown it less for its looks—and, to be fair, it is a weedy, if satisfyingly green, thing—than for the food it put on their tables.

Purslane is a plant of mysterious origins. It would seem to be native to the Middle East, though some archaeological evidence suggests that it arrived in the New World before Columbus, a matter that scholars are puzzling over even now. Whatever the case, it is well adapted to many climates, growing in many very different environments around the world. That ubiquity and variability, unfortunately for purslane's reputation, is yet more evidence that the plant is a weed, strictly speaking; in some places where native plants have been compromised, it's even an invasive weed, crowding out the indigenes and considered noxious as a result. Still, like basil, verdolaga produces chemicals that most insects seem not to like, with the result that it has few insect pests. Most animals seem not to prefer it, either, making it a good plant to grow on the edges of gardens where hungry critters come to browse.

The plant contains abundant omega–3 fatty acids of the kind found in fish, flax seeds, and a few other dietary sources. It also contains significant amounts of vitamins A and C, as well as calcium, iron, magnesium, potassium, and cancer-fighting antioxidants. Unlike fish, the most usual source of those fatty acids, it does not contain mercury. Artemis Simopoulos, a medical researcher, found a clump of purslane growing, conveniently, alongside a sidewalk just outside his office at the National Institutes of Health in Washington, DC, and conducted a chemical analysis, discovering that purslane contains enough vitamin E to fulfill the recommended daily requirement in a single serving, while its base fatty acid, alpha-linolenic, is found in concentrations up to fifteen times higher than in lettuce, its most common dietary source outside of fish.

On top of all that, purslane, like spinach, contains an abundance of oxalates. This means that it should be eaten in moderation by anyone susceptible to kidney stones—a common malady in the desert, of course, where the water is dense with minerals—but plentifully by everyone else. It also seems to help control cholesterol and is often used in poultry feed to lower cholesterol in eggs. An added bonus is that its mix of soluble and insoluble fibers helps clean out your system in several ways, making it an ideal addition to weight-loss diets.

As verdolaga, common purslane is something for which Mexicans outside of Mexico are known to pine. In Durango, it's often eaten with pork. In southern Arizona, I've had it fried with chiles and onions and eaten on fried tortillas with a smear of beans and white cheese, as if a distant cousin of an Italian pizza margarita. Like the chimichanga, that version is slowly spreading to restaurants outside the region with deep menus or extensive vegetarian offerings. I haven't yet seen it in Texas, though I have seen menudo there, a beloved Sonoran/Arizona hangover remedy making judicious use of onions, hominy, broth, the red-hot peppers called chiltepines, and tripe.

I have been writing as if, between the states and microregions of the Southwest, there were culinary barriers as tall and sinister as the steel walls separating Mexico from various American ports of entry. There are no such things, and, naturally enough, people cross the boundaries of regional differences just as easily as they cross the boundaries of regions—or those ludicrous walls, for that matter. People from Zacatecas marry people from Sonora and move to Tucson. Their children marry the children of people from all over the world and move to Los Angeles, Chicago, Zurich. They share recipes, and in time they make new traditions.

In his novel *La Maravilla*, a work of art as fine as its name, the Arizona-born writer Alfredo Véa recounts the women of his protagonist's family

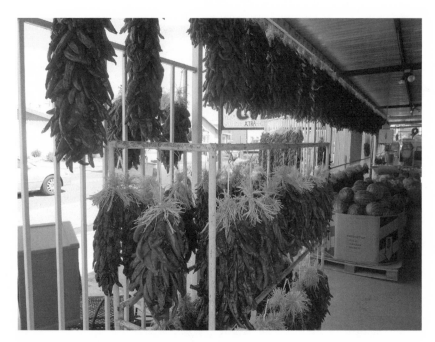

Chile ristras for sale in Hatch, New Mexico, ground zero for chile production in the Southwest.

making salsa. Arizonans, as we have said, eat beef—but here, at home, we find them eating a stew of beef and pork, mixing the proclivities of Arizona and New Mexico and not feeling the slightest bit guilty for it. The meat has been simmering on the stovetop for hours and hours, while the salsa has been curing for days, a huge pot cooking on an open fire for the extra smokiness of the wood. Writes Véa, the women in the kitchen "had turned the red chiles on the embers till the skins pulled away easily. Then the red flesh had been ground by hand on the stone *metate* along with the potent seeds. Garlic cloves followed the chile into the *metate*. To the garlic and chile were added a bit of broth from the meat pot, some sifted Gold Medal flour, and a handful of oregano." And perhaps not just any oregano, but Mexican oregano, or verbena, a flavor subtly distinct from its Mediterranean cousin.

Those simple ingredients, plus long practice, are enough for us to make fine salsas of our own, but there are secrets in each cook's preparation. Virginia Vasquez, the lead chef in Véa's tale, employed two: the chiles came from a little market across the line in Mexico, and they were cooked in beat-up old pots that had been serving her in her kitchen for decades. As Virginia, the "keeper of the chiles," says to her hungry family, "It takes no effort to be loyal to something that serves you so well and so long."

The right tools, the right ingredients, the right knowledge: On these things all that is human turns and nowhere more artfully than in the kitchen. Each kitchen is different, loyal to its own secrets and traditions, and it is from that as much as from local ingredients that regional variations are born. For a pan-Southwestern meal, then, try a range of courses: guacamole from California avocados, a carne asada taco from Arizona, a bowl of red from Texas, rice and beans and cabbage and all the fixings, and then top it off with a specialty of New Mexico and New Mexico alone, the wonder that is the sopapilla, a square of dough deep-fried until it puffs up, then served with honey and perhaps a dusting of sugar and cinnamon.

There are other regional preferences and differences. Tortillas in Arizona seem to be generally thinner than those in New Mexico and California. Vegetable dishes turn up on more California menus than in Texas. Then there is the matter of tamales, traditionally made with pork or beef—for chicken tends to dry up when entombed in masa, though legs hold up better than breasts. Farther south in Mexico banana leaves take the place of corn husks, and mole negro—a blend of chocolate and pepper—takes the place of salsa, but it is unsafe to generalize much beyond that. In Acapulco, for instance, you might find a tamale filled with shrimp, but so might you in Houston. In Santa Fe the tamale might be made with blue corn. In Tucson the green corn tamale has long been a specialty, made of masa studded with moist kernels of corn and filled with chiles and white cheese; traditionally, green corn tamales were served only in summertime, but that has given way to their enjoyment year round. And in Los Angeles Sonoran vendors were selling tamales from wheeled carts when Anglos first arrived. Writing in 1897, a transplant to California named Corinne Updegraff tried to describe one of the things for the readers of *Munsey's Magazine* back East:

An Eastern tamale is a Frankfurter in the middle of a roll; a Western tamale, the kind you buy from a dusky, dark eyed Spaniard, or a Mexican boy, who stands by the side of his little wagon on a cold night, and shivers in the glimmering light of a dim lantern until the theaters are out and his stock is disposed of—that is quite a different thing. Paste is not more widely different from diamonds than are the Eastern sausage rolls from the steaming corn husks wrapped around a mixture of meal and butter and chicken and olives and red peppers, with special reference to the red peppers. But a tamale cannot be described, it has to be appreciated.

Outside of Mexico, tamales were a very strictly Southwestern thing until the twentieth century. Leave Texas and its cultural outposts, and you were not likely to encounter one by that name anywhere else. One such outpost was western Arkansas, where a teenage girl named Mattie Ross, the protagonist of Charles Portis's great novel *True Grit*, encounters one in 1875: "A noisy boy was going through the crowd selling parched peanuts and fudge. Another one was selling 'hot tamales' out of a bucket. This is a cornmeal tube filled with spicy meat that they eat in Old Mexico. They are not bad."

No, they are not bad, though, like everything else, they can be bad for you. The distinguished scholar of *chicanismo* Rodolfo Acuña, a Californian of Sonoran descent, recalls, "When I was a child I remember my mother, grandmother and aunts making tamales. They prepared the masa dipping into a huge tin can full of pork lard. Today canola and/or corn oil has been substituted for the lard even though connoisseurs tell me that the tamales don't taste the same." He adds, wryly, "My wife, however, is a health nut and won't even use corn oil because of the potential for GMO contamination." Tamales with canola oil, served with cold water or fruit juice instead of beer—well, all things change, change brought about, as Acuña wisely says, "by making ethical choices and forcing people to choose what they value the most."

However and wherever it is cooked, a tamale is a wondrous thing, and tamales have traveled all through the Southwest and beyond for centuries. We will never have an exact genealogy, just as we will never know exactly where one Mexican food frontier in the Southwest begins and another ends. It's one of our more pleasant duties, though, to try to map out that geography from kitchen to kitchen and hearth and hearth, on the trail of the elusive bowl of red and the last of the red-hot burritos.

5. **The Anglo Frontier**

Daniel Boone did not wear a coonskin cap.

The legend of the American frontier is in large part the legend of Daniel Boone, who, more than any other single individual, opened the Southwest to Anglo settlement. His name conjures the image of a gaunt, buckskin-clad warrior, possibly grappling with a fierce Indian or dispatching a grizzly, doing anything but sitting still. That Boone would be a simple man, someone who lived to kill bears and Indians, able to sound out only a few words of the family Bible—and very quick to go for his gun if he felt that he needed to shoot you for some reason or another.

As is so often the case, however, the Daniel Boone of folklore is not the Daniel Boone of history.

Daniel was born on October 22, 1734, the son of Quakers who had left their native England and moved to Pennsylvania. In 1750 the Boones relocated to a farmstead on the Yadkin River in North Carolina, and sixteen-year-old Daniel became a professional hunter, working the Appalachian Mountains for months at a time.

Most European emigrants to the United States had little knowledge of hunting, which was reserved for the nobility. In Europe, wherever there was a patch of land big enough to sustain a population of wild animals, the chances were good that those animals and that land belonged to some baron or earl or lord, if not the king himself. A successful hunter out on the American frontier would have stood out from most people for his knowledge of guns and how to use them. If he were to have any longevity, that frontier hunter would have to acquire some knowledge of Indian languages and customs, making him an intermediary between Europe and Native America and enhancing his status even more. Such a hunter would have been a necessary, useful figure—and a good friend to have out in the backcountry.

Daniel Boone acquired all these skills. So proficient a backwoodsman was he that the British Army pressed him into service in the French and Indian War alongside another American who would soon enter the history books—George Washington. The Virginia gentleman, sad to say, wasn't much of a soldier in those days. French prisoners of war were executed on Washington's watch, and when the news got out, the rest of the French army and their Indian allies hit back hard, wiping out a British command under General Edward Braddock. Washington and Boone both had to flee far away from the frontier in order to save their skins.

Washington stayed away from the deep Appalachians for the rest of his life, but in 1773 Daniel Boone led his family to Kentucky. When the American Revolution came three years later, he was accused of being pro-British—yet, as soon as the opportunity arose, he was appointed a colonel in the militia. Following another disastrous battle, he was court-martialed but acquitted, and after the war he kept his rank while serving as both a representative in the Virginia assembly and county sheriff at home in Kentucky, elected to both posts by a landslide.

In 1784 John Filson, a Pennsylvania schoolteacher, published a thoroughly romanticized book called *The Discovery, Settlement and Present State of Kentucke*, in which Boone starred as a tough, quick-tempered Indian fighter, though still without a coonskin cap. The book was translated into several European languages, and the great German poet Johann Wolfgang von Goethe held Daniel Boone up as the model of the Swiss philosopher Jean-Jacques Rousseau's "natural man," while Lord Byron devoted a section of his epic poem *Don Juan* to the frontiersman, calling Boone "happiest of mortals any where."

He was a great hunter and explorer, but in other pursuits he was less accomplished. He often worked as a surveyor for land companies, traveling as far as eastern Texas in their service. But he wasn't very good at it, and his maps were seldom accurate. Neither was he much of a businessman; at one point he owned more than a hundred thousand acres of land, but he lost most of it to swindlers. Boone later remarked to a visiting journalist that "while he could never with safety repose confidence in a Yankee, he had never been deceived by any Indian, and he should certainly prefer a state of nature to a state of civilization."

Death claimed Daniel Boone on September 26, 1820, at the age of eighty-five, at his home in Missouri, which had been a Spanish colony when he left the United States and moved there in 1799. After that, scarcely a decade went by when some new biography or novel featuring Boone did not appear, each adding a new tall tale. In my time, people learned of Boone through the immensely popular television show that ran from 1964 to 1970, in which Fess Parker, who liked the costumes, simply repeated his portrayal of Davy Crockett in an earlier Walt Disney movie, making the peaceful Boone "the rippin'est, roarin'est, fightin'est man the frontier ever knew," putting a coonskin cap on him in the bargain, and extending the legend even further from the far more interesting truth.

I have spent so much time talking about Daniel Boone because Daniel Boone was the definitive creature of the American frontier, creator of the frontier and created by the frontier. But what was that frontier? And where was it?

By definition, a frontier is something that is in front: a sort of no-man's-land that divides us from them. The word is Latin in origin, dating to the time of the early Roman Empire, and meaning the territory that lay between the limits of that Empire and the beginning of the savage territory that was Germany.

Two thousand and one years ago, in 9 CE, a Roman general named Publius Quinctilius Varus led a mighty army made up of three Roman legions across the Rhine River into the Teutoburg Forest in what is now northwestern Germany. There he was attacked by a larger force of Germanic tribespeople, many of whom had at one time or another served in the Roman army and knew its tactics inside and out. It was the Roman Little Big Horn: all twenty thousand of those Roman soldiers died in the massacre that followed, and thereafter it was official Roman policy not to even try to conquer Germany.

Edward Braddock's forces suffered their own Teutoburg Forest in the slaughter that took place near what is now Pittsburgh, Pennsylvania, the fight that sent Washington and Boone running. For the next decade, it was official British policy to keep east of the Appalachian Mountains. The Proclamation of 1763 forbade all white settlement on Indian territory, ordered those settlers already there to withdraw, and strictly limited future settlement away from the coast. For the first time in the history of European colonization in the New World, the proclamation recognized Indian land titles, and in doing so it put up a big no trespassing sign telling English subjects to keep their distance from the interior of North America.

The frontier became, if you'll forgive the word, the backtier. It was the backyard in which the children of England were forbidden to play, the very limits of Britain, even as the Spanish and French were active far beyond the mountains. For a time, that policy kept the English colonists from spilling over the Appalachians, apart from a few headstrong and daring people such as Daniel Boone. They had to content themselves with building farms and towns and cities east of the great peaks.

Edmund Burke, the great English political theorist, knew that people like Boone would eventually defy the law and settle in what he called the "desert." He warned of the effects of letting them travel west: "Already they have topped the Appalachian mountains," he wrote in 1770. "From thence they behold before them an immense plain, one vast, rich, level meadow; a square of five hundred miles. Over this they would wander without possibility of restraint; they would change their manners with their habits of life; they would soon forget a government by which they were disowned; would become hordes of English Tartars, pouring down upon your unfortified frontiers a fierce and irresistible cavalry."

The English, in other words, once confronting the space and freedom of the frontier, would become Indians. And that is just what happened: Throughout American history, those on the frontier have tended to appropriate Native American dress, customs, and habits, to become not English or Indian but something in between, a third culture. This is what happens on borders: people from one culture meet people from another culture, and in time they become a third culture, neither one nor the other. That is one reason why Arizonans are a touch different from people in, say, Massachusetts.

Roast Venison

My friend and high school classmate Scott Leysath moved to the Southwest about the time I did, and there he learned the fine arts of fine cooking. He has since operated and owned restaurants in California and become well known as the Sporting Chef, advising hunters, cooks, and diners on how to secure and prepare wild game. Here are his thoughts on cooking venison:

> The biggest mistake that most home cooks make when cooking venison is to overcook it. Considering that a deer steak is roughly ten times leaner than a comparable cut of beef, it is much less forgiving when cooked past medium-rare, or about 135 degrees at the center. Of course, like beef, different cuts of venison require cooking methods best suited to specific muscle groups. Tough cuts from the shoulders, necks, and shanks are best braised at low temperature for several hours until tender. Tenderloins, loins, and the better hindquarter muscles should be prepared with high heat for just a few minutes per side.

> To prepare a proper venison steak, remove all gristle, sinew, and connective tissue. Rub with olive oil and apply a liberal amount of coarse salt and pepper. Place on a grill over white-hot coals or in a medium-hot heavy skillet. Brown on one side, flip over and cook the other side for only 2 to 3 minutes, depending on the thickness of the steak, but not past medium-rare. Venison pairs well with earthy sautéed mushrooms and a full-bodied red wine.

It is also the reason that Southwestern food is different from other food.

Massachusetts was once a frontier, and it is no accident that the perpetrators of the Boston Tea Party donned Indian headdresses before sending British cargo into the drink; they at once wanted to disguise themselves and proclaim a kind of kinship with the continent's first inhabitants. England became a *them* for the American colonists, and the Indians became an *us*. Dressing in Indian dress allowed the New England Puritans to enjoy freedoms that would not have been possible in plain-spun black tunics. The Puritans were not the only ones to seize on the possibilities of this freedom. There were the Boy Scouts, for instance, whose American founder, Ernest Thompson Seton, reveled in the freedom that he imagined Indians enjoyed, even if he suspected real Indians of harboring "unpatriotic sentiments." One southern Colorado Boy Scout troop took this literally. They went so far native that the boys ran away and lived in the forest, and it took months to round them up and send them to the reservations of their bedrooms. While they were on the loose, though, these young men of La Junta managed to reconstruct the secret Shalako ceremony of the Zuni Indians so convincingly that Zuni elders built a special kiva for the masks the scouts had made.

In 1675, in New England, English settlers and Algonquian Indians fought a bitter guerrilla war that lasted for eighteen months. By proportion of population, King Philip's War inflicted greater casualties than any other war in American history, and with more than the usual atrocities: men, women, even children were tortured and murdered on both sides, and whole cities were burned to the ground.

King Philip's War is riddled with mysteries. The English, half a century removed from their ancestral homeland, had adopted Native American customs and cuisine, had stopped attending church, had moved farther and farther inland, away from European settlements. The Indians, for their part, had taken to wearing clothes, living in houses, and reading the Bible. With identities thus confused, each side waged a war that the other condemned as brutal and savage, and thousands of people died in the bargain.

Back in Europe, the people were no strangers to bitter wars that hinged on cultural differences and that resulted in thousands of deaths.

Even so, apart from those who could afford to build castles, people lived more or less in the open. Traditional villages were self-sufficient and self-contained, with people pitching in and doing what needed to be done, sharing chores and tools, with the occasional beggar or traveling peddler passing through to bring news of the outside world. The fields were small and unfenced. They were scattered around the village, and they were usually the property of some nobleman or another who received rents for the privilege of someone else's farming the fields.

In America it was different. Fields were typically owned, not rented. They were single, not scattered. And there were no peasants as such to pitch in and help each other bring in the crops. Neighbors were useful when it came to fighting off Indian attacks but necessary nuisances at other times, and

Americans expressed their attitude with what was a comparative rarity in Europe: a wall or fence to keep those neighbors away.

English observers of the American scene were puzzled by what one correspondent called "a mania for enclosures." Another London paper commented, "The stripping of forests to build fortifications around personal property is a perfect example of the way those people in the New World live and think." Life must have been very dangerous, one would think, for such protections to have become necessary, but it really wasn't: If fences were used only for military reasons in the Old World, in the New World they proclaimed, "This land and this stuff are mine." Fences did away with the need for the hired shepherd, a rarity in the New World. With fences, you did not need to keep an eye on your animals, because they could not wander far, or on your neighbors' animals, which could not wander in and eat your garden.

Consequently, East of the Mississippi, calculated an Iowa agricultural census in the mid-nineteenth century, six million miles of boards took the form of wooden fences. How the census arrived at the calculation is very hard to say. If we accept the figure as accurate, the cost of those fences in those days would have been nearly $2 billion—about the size of the national debt in the years just before the Civil War, which indicates just how important keeping our possessions from others was to us.

All of these stories figure into the story of the American frontier, which includes the Southwest, a region won partly by conquest and partly by checkbook.

The frontier opened at the end of the Revolutionary War, when the provisions of the hated Proclamation of 1763 were scrapped. By that time, more than one hundred thousand Americans were already living west of the Appalachian Mountains. Within a few years, towns like Nashville and Cincinnati were founded, as hundreds of thousands of new settlers pushed across the Appalachians and into the valleys of the Ohio and Mississippi Rivers. By 1820 the frontier had moved well into what was called the Old Northwest, into Illinois and Michigan. By 1830 it had crossed the Mississippi. By 1840 the land organized as states was smaller than the land organized as territories, and the states began to argue over whether slavery would be allowed into this new country. The argument grew fiercer as the years wore on. By 1850 when the frontier had bypassed the Rocky Mountains, the western Great Plains, and the

Southwest, which were full of uncooperative Indians, and jumped straight to California and Alaska, the argument about slavery turned into the beginnings of the Civil War.

In 1893, three years after the superintendent of the census announced that the Western frontier was closed, Frederick Jackson Turner, a historian from the University of Wisconsin, advanced a thesis that the conquest of that frontier had given American society its special character. Western expansion, he said, accounted for Americans' optimism, their rugged independence, and their stress on adaptability, ingenuity, and self-reliance. The frontier, in other words, had created a nation of Daniel Boones.

The thesis overlooked a crucial fact: The settlement of the West was not an individual matter. It never had been. It had depended all along on intervention by the federal government. The federal government had dispatched explorers to survey the region and cavalry units to confine Native Americans to reservations. Thomas Jefferson had wanted to extend the agricultural zones of his native Virginia westward, writing, "I think we shall be virtuous as long as agriculture is our principal object, which will be the case, while there remains vacant lands in any part of America. When we get piled upon one another in large cities, as in Europe, we shall become corrupt." Jefferson had recommended that the federal lands of the West be given away to ordinary people, since those lands cost almost nothing—his government, after all, had paid only $15 million, about $250 million in today's money, for the vast territory called the Louisiana Purchase, a sum that Jefferson had been prepared to pay France just for the port of New Orleans alone.

But that's not the way it worked out. Instead, for most of the nineteenth century, the frontier lands were sold off in 640-acre parcels, not to individuals but to the railroads and other corporations, which then turned around and sold them in smaller parcels to farmers, ranchers, and other settlers. Not surprisingly, the corporations that made out best were the ones that contributed money to the campaigns of the most influential members of Congress. The government used the money to retire debt, the corporations to grow rich. It was a happy arrangement all around, made uncomfortable only when reformers, historians, and journalists came around. When thinking of the history of the American Southwest, in short, do not think of John Wayne in *The Man Who Shot Liberty Valance*, but of Lionel Barrymore in *It's a Wonderful Life*.

The corporate argument held that the original inhabitants of the newly

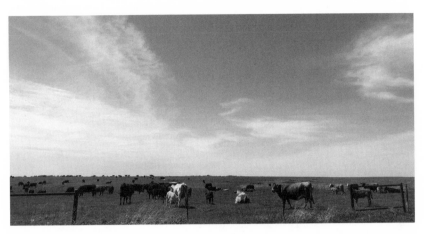

The Great Plains, settled by corporations and the government.

acquired lands were little more than inconveniences. "Since the time of the Puritans in early seventeenth-century Massachusetts," writes historian Michael Green, "Europeans and Anglo-Americans had constructed an argument to justify the taking of Indian land that rested on the idea that commercial agriculture, with its privately owned parcels of land, plows, fences, and livestock and its production of surplus crops, was morally superior to the lifeways of Native Americans. Europeans and their American descendants often described the Indians as wandering hunters who refused to subdue and develop their land. They would not credit the agricultural subsistence base of nearly all eastern Native societies because in those societies women were the farmers. Believing that the important work of society was done by men, they defined Indian societies by what men did." Because women were the landholders, the workers of the land, and in many cases the political and economic heads of the households to which they belonged, these Indian societies simply did not count—and therefore, the newcomers had no pressing need to reckon them in any kind of moral calculus, particularly one whose overarching goal was the acquisition of new land and of the wealth that grew from it.

Edmund Burke's English Tartars materialized almost as soon as the frontier opened. These backcountry Americans wanted to do as they pleased without suffering being told what to do: they wanted to shoot whatever game they cared to, cut down whatever forests they cared to, sink mines into whatever mountains they cared to, and they bitterly resented it when any government told them otherwise. They formed ragtag armies to express that resentment. In frontier New York they were called "cowboys," and during the Revolutionary War they fought against British and Continental forces alike. In frontier South Carolina they were called the Regulators, the ancestors of the Texas Rangers and other vigilante outfits, and rode around hanging suspected criminals and troublemakers and advising strangers to move on. As the frontier moved, the Regulators and the cowboys moved: these are the men who brought us the Alamo and the War with Mexico, the Sand Creek Massacre and the Skeleton Cave Massacre, the men who kept on pushing west until there was no more west to push to.

Culturally, the Southwest was—and, with exception of California and northern New Mexico, remains—an extension of the South, a place to which Southerners moved after the land was played out back home. Edmund Ruffin, the fiery secessionist who fired the first shot at Fort Sumter, observed that "the great error of southern agriculture is the general practice of exhausting culture—the almost universal deterioration of the productive power of the soil, which power is the main and essential foundation of all agricultural wealth." For footloose Southerners, it was natural to press on once this deterioration was evident.

Texas, the first of the Southwestern lands to receive these Anglo newcomers, looked to Memphis and New Orleans as its natural capitals, supplied from both. An Irish immigrant named Oliver Pollock had established a commercial empire in the latter city in the first years of the new American republic, acting as an intermediary between Spanish, French, and American interests, selling sugar, rum, coffee, and other goods to travelers into the interior. He recalled, "I supplied dry goods from London, Negroes from Africa, and flour from Philadelphia," linking the Gulf Coast to the larger world economy.

All the colonies of British North America permitted slavery but to varying degrees of economic importance. Though legalized in Massachusetts in 1641, slavery was little practiced in New England, a predominantly Puritan region of small farms and cities. Where the piedmont broadened and the soil became less stony, the population of slaves—most, though not all, from West Africa by the beginning of the eighteenth century—grew steadily over the years. The greatest slave-trading center in the colonies was the Quaker center of Philadelphia, where a young printer named Benjamin Franklin grew wealthy publishing notices of slave auctions, but by far the largest population of slaves lived in Virginia and the Carolinas, the places where those large royalist estates, soon to become known as plantations, were established and large numbers of field workers were needed to bring in crops of maize, cotton, and tobacco bound for eager ports in the British Isles and elsewhere in Europe.

By the time of the American Revolution, slavery was waning everywhere but the South. And after the Revolution, when British royal prohibitions against settling west of the Appalachians were no longer in force, numerous questions came to the forefront: How would the western reaches of North America, the territories beyond the Mississippi, be settled? Would they be extensions of existing states, as Kentucky was of Virginia and Tennessee of North Carolina, or would they be federal domains, or would they be self-governing entities from the start? And most importantly, would slavery be permitted in these new lands, or would it be prohibited?

The questions of states' rights and western expansion that arose in the years of the early republic and roiled in the early decades of the nineteenth century were all, in some way, contingent on the underlying reality of slavery. Apologists for the secession today who like to insist that the Civil War of the 1860s was not about slavery but about the rights of independent states versus the federated nation are partly right: For some Southerners, slavery was secondary to the ability of Georgia, say, to determine what laws it would uphold and suppress.

Still, slavery touched on and underlay all those questions, and so it was that when people from the northern states pressed westward, to places like Ohio and Illinois, they tended to settle in farms owned by freeholders, while when the cavaliers and borderers of the southern tier pressed westward, they looked at the hot, seemingly empty lands of Texas and beyond as the future homes of huge farms and ranches best staffed by enslaved people. When Texas became independent—and one reason that the settlers from the South who arrived there broke away from Mexico is that slavery was illegal in the former Spanish colony—the Southerners looked farther west still, imagining a slave empire that stretched all the way to the Pacific Ocean. The agriculture that they established in Texas, with great fields of food crops but also of cotton and tobacco, was not big simply because the place was big but because an army of workers would be on hand to plant it, harvest it, process it, and bring it to market.

Push beyond the agriculturally congenial coastal plain of Texas, move east from the thin Mediterranean coast of California, and leave the narrow well-watered river valleys of the interior, and you are in dry, vast country best suited to one kind of agriculture above all others: livestock grazing.

Cattle had roamed the arid lands of New Spain since the 1500s, taking the place of the Pleistocene browsers that had been driven extinct many thousands of years earlier. In the Spanish period, their herds tended to be small except in well-watered, grassy southern California, where the biblical "cattle on a thousand hills" was more than a poetic convention. The Americans who arrived in the Southwest had different ideas: they believed that bigger was better and that the new country was too big to fail, unlike those exhausted Southern lands they had left behind. Sylvester Mowry, an entrepreneur who worked out of Tucson and ran afoul of Union troops there for his Confederate sympathies, launched a campaign to convince Texas cattlemen to relocate to Arizona. The new territorial governor, a Union man, rejoined, "the sun never shone on better grazing country," glossing over the fact that much of it was rocky, cactus-strewn desert.

In 1870 there were perhaps five thousand head of cattle in the Arizona Territory. In 1872 a self-made livestock producer named Henry Hooker established a huge new spread in southeastern Arizona. Hooker and other ranchers brought in vast herds from Texas, and by 1890 there were about a million and a half cattle in Arizona, their meat in constant demand in markets in the eastern United States and Europe. Just a couple of years after that, the number of cattle in Arizona doubled again, and even as everyone in America, it seemed, ate thick steaks three meals a day, the desert began to reel from the effects of overgrazing, as the cattle ate every bit of vegetation they happened upon. Still, the ranches kept growing, with spreads like the XIT Ranch of northern Texas and the Hashknife of northern Arizona taking in millions of acres.

The same logarithmic growth had marked the cattle industry in Texas. In 1867 about thirty-five thousand head were driven from Texas to the railhead in Abilene, Kansas. Four years later, after the transcontinental railroad was finished, the figure had jumped to nearly three quarters of a million. But that number represents only the cattle driven to distant markets, for within Texas during the Civil War years there were at least three million and probably as many as five million head of cattle in herds so large that they were effectively too big to be controlled—and thus, after a fashion, were wild, the root meaning of the old Spanish cattle term *criollo*, their number adding to the vast herds of feral pigs and wild horses that roamed the border country.

Two things turned the cattle boom around. In 1892 and 1893 the American economy weathered a terrible depression, throwing millions of people out of work, disintegrating fortunes, and putting an end to the availability of cheap beef in every corner of the country. At the same time, a huge drought settled in on the Southwest. O'odham shamans had predicted apocalyptic effects when the cattle first arrived, a time when a massive earthquake struck northwestern Mexico and rattled throughout southern California and Arizona. Now their words seemed to be coming true, as unacclimated cattle from introduced English stock keeled over in the heat; it was said that a person could skip a rock from one carcass to another across the entire Southwest. By 1895 somewhere between half and two-thirds of all the cattle in the region had died off, and people went with them, whole counties being effectively abandoned as their inhabitants returned to wetter country to the east.

By 1900 the rains were beginning to return and with them the cattle industry, which even today has political clout that is disproportionate to its actual position in the Southwestern economy. And even today we think of the rancher and the longhorn as being iconic figures of the region—not for nothing was John Wayne, the actor, also an investor in Southwestern livestock and for a time the owner of an Arizona cattle company and one of the largest private feedlots in the United States in the 1950s.

The tale of one young cowboy is particularly instructive here. Beginning in the 1860s Lincoln County, New Mexico, where the southernmost stretches of the Rocky Mountains meet the first hints of the Great Plains, was unlike most other places in the region in being oddly violent. There were Apache raids, crimes fanned by ethnic tensions between Anglos and Hispanics, and a business rivalry that would lead to the so-called Lincoln County War.

Into this scene arrived a young man named William Bonney, born sometime between 1857 and 1860 in New York City, far from the frontier. The son of Irish immigrants who had fled the Potato Famine, his given name was

Henry McCarty. In 1873 his widowed mother married another Irish settler, William Antrim, and her son took his stepfather's name. The new family moved west to Santa Fe, then Silver City, seeking fortune in New Mexico.

But the older Antrim and his wife died of the flu, and Henry was on his own. He turned to petty crime, finally running away from the equivalent of a juvenile detention center to Arizona, where he found work as a ranch hand in the pay of none other than Henry Hooker. The older wranglers liked "the Kid," as they called him, and he was useful in that he spoke good Spanish and worked without complaint, helping out with the chuck wagon as the herds moved across the desert and enduring the taunts of his fellows, who scornfully called cooks "biscuit-shooters," "bean-masters," and "pot rustlers" but ate what they were served up all the same.

In 1877 following an altercation that led to his shooting a blowhard on the Hooker spread, Henry went east, arriving in Lincoln under the new name of Sam H. Bonney. It was a fraught time. Hispanic farmers, along with Anglos who married into Mexican families, had not only Apache raiders to fear but also racist Southern vigilantes who would have been Klansmen back home. Farmers of any kind, who were in the habit of putting up fences, were hunted by ranchers, who hated the inconvenience those fences caused their cattle. Guns may have been rarely deployed elsewhere on the frontier, but not in Lincoln.

More distant, but just as worrisome, was a cabal of businessmen based in Santa Fe informally called "the Ring," whose corrupting influence over politics and business alike would become infamous over the course of several generations and would produce sideshows such as the Teapot Dome scandal half a century later. Two of Lincoln's most prosperous merchants, J. J. Dolan and L. G. Murphy, were friendly with the Ring, and they were locked in rivalry against a rancher named John Chisum over the control of southern New Mexico's cattle industry and all that came with it: banking, real estate, mercantile commerce, and the railroad.

The story becomes still more complex. Young William Bonney, as he was now known, went to work for an ally of Chisum's, a British immigrant named John Tunstall, himself just barely twenty-four years old. One day members of a Lincoln County sheriff's posse, led by Dolan, ambushed and murdered Tunstall. Billy Bonney found the body and swore out a complaint against Dolan. The constable, Atanasio Martinez, deputized Billy, and they went to

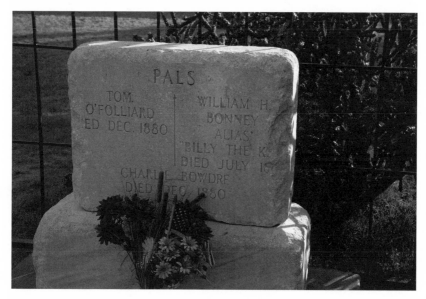

The grave of Billy the Kid in Fort Sumner, New Mexico.

serve Dolan's arrest warrant at Murphy's store. When they arrived, the county sheriff, who was in cahoots with The Ring, arrested them instead.

Eventually they were released and Billy joined with other Tunstall ranch hands in a ten-man vigilante force called—yes, the Regulators. They began hunting down members of the sheriff's posse and killing them one by one, a vendetta that went on until midsummer and left dozens of men dead on both sides, including the sheriff. Many innocent civilians were caught in the cross-fire, and the bloodshed continued unabated even after President Rutherford B. Hayes removed the corrupt territorial governor and replaced him with General Lew Wallace, a Civil War hero whose famous novel *Ben-Hur* was published a few months later. For more than a year, Wallace tried to convince Billy Bonney to give himself up so that he might testify in court against the Dolan-Murphy faction. When Billy was finally arrested in March 1879, however, he was not allowed to speak. Instead he was charged with the sheriff's murder, which he swore he had not committed. He was sentenced to hang, but he somehow managed to escape.

Late in the evening of July 14, 1881, a lawman named Pat Garrett crept into the room where Bonney lay sleeping. He must have made a noise, for the Kid

Corn Dodgers

Laura Gayle Wilson arrived in Texas in the early 1850s and settled down to ranch life in the Hill Country. In 1853 she jotted down a recipe that she transmitted to a ranch cook, saying that the resulting corn dodgers "will keep several days in a saddle bag."

About 2 cups cornmeal, ⅔ teaspoon salt, and enough boiling water so you can pick them up and make a patty (about like a mud patty you made as a child).

These may also be made on a clean shovel at the edge of a campfire. Be sure they are brown on both sides.

She later recalled, "These cakes and black coffee made in a tin can on a fire kept many a cowboy going on the long trail rides to the railroad."

sprang to his feet and called out "*¿Quien es? ¿Quien es?*" That is, "Who is it? Who is it?"—there were no English-only laws on the frontier. Garrett replied by firing twice. One bullet struck the unarmed Bonney in the chest, and he died instantly.

Henry McCarty. Henry Antrim. Billy Antrim. The Kid. Kid Antrim. Billy Bonney. Billy the Kid. A Catholic defender of Hispanics on a Protestant frontier, a man who, like Kit Carson, preferred chile colorado to any other meal.

Conrad Richter's 1937 novel *Sea of Grass* catches some of the reverberations of a ring that had become a triangle in the years following the death of Billy the Kid. At one corner is Jim Brewton, a wealthy cattle rancher who enjoys near-absolute power in his domain—and knows it, even as he knows his empire will soon pass. At the beginning of the novel, his vast ranch, set somewhere near where the Rio Puerco joins the Rio Grande in central New Mexico, has been "quartered . . . like a steer on the meat block," its glory days fifty years gone.

At another corner is Brewton's wife, Lutie, who, at the beginning of the book, has come to the rough-and-tumble frontier town of Salt Fork with very high hopes for a better life. It is evident soon enough that she will be disappointed, for Lutie is untamable, as is the land, and Jim Brewton is in the business of subduing whatever stands before him—including his neighbors, the despised "nesters," settlers who fence the land in order to keep their crops safe and thus keep the cattle baron's herds from traveling wherever they will. The ensuing struggle for control of the land often turns violent, as Brewton allows when recalling one former neighbor who "was not run off because he wanted to settle those hundred and sixty acres"—a homestead allotment, that is—"but because of what he wanted to do with the land."

What he wanted to do with the land was grow something other than cattle, of course. The nesters have a defender in the district attorney, Brice Chamberlain, who confronts Brewton early on, asking him whether he might not be persuaded to turn over some of his million-acre-plus domain to the newcomers. Brewton is unmoved. "I have sympathy for the pioneer settler who came out here and risked his life and family among the Indians," he thunders. "And I hope I have a little charity for the nester who waited until the country was safe and peaceable before he filed a homestead on someone else's range who fought for it." Nonetheless, he adds, he has no truck with the nester who would plow up the best grazing land for miles in a land too dry to farm—and he will drive out the first who tries to do so, and the last.

Brewton and Chamberlain's feud implicates Lutie in ways that sensitive readers of Richter's era must have found shocking. And it carries on into the next generation, when the cattle ranchers lose their influence as the farmers gain more and more land and with it more and more political dominance. Drought soon settles in on the land and proves Brewton right, just as drought and poor farming practices turned much of the Southwest into a Dust Bowl in the era in which Richter's book appeared. As the topsoil disappears, as the sea of grass dies, and as all he has worked for disintegrates all around him, proud but broken Jim Brewton turns out to be perhaps the most sympathetic character in the book—certainly more so than Chamberlain, who, we learn, has had other motives for his championship of the little man for all those years.

The Indian Wars, ethnic strife, and the violence of cattlemen versus nesters notwithstanding, if you were an Anglo, at least, the frontier was not a particularly dangerous place to be. For every Western gunfighter there were a thousand merchants and a hundred restaurants, for every outlaw ten thousand farmers. In cities like Denver, Santa Fe, and Abilene very few citizens owned guns or had need to. The decades-long war against Native America was being staged in remote corners of the country, and, as for bad men, few but the local tall-tale spinner had ever seen one.

In 1890, nine years after Billy the Kid died, the superintendent of the US Census announced that the West was filling up so fast that "there can hardly be said to be a frontier line." In just a quarter century, the frontier had been settled. Three million families started farms on the Great Plains during these years. The Indian Wars over, New Mexico and Arizona were teeming with Anglo newcomers. So were Colorado, Montana, Utah, and the states of the Pacific Coast. As they came, those people staked out what was theirs, fiercely defending their little empires against their neighbors. Consequently, the open frontier, the land of wide-open spaces, was crisscrossed with fences.

They built walls and streets and houses, too. Though we like to think of the West as a rural place, by 1890 most of the West's population lived in cities—the most urbanized region in the country, just as it is today. That's not the story that most of us learned in our history books, which favor a more heroic, more individualistic view of things in the place of the tangled history of the frontier, one marked by ambition and greed, by power brokering and wheeling and dealing, and by the contributions and hard work and good citizenship of many people from all over the world, about which more to come.

Food was scarce on the early Southwestern frontier. According to a migrant named Joel Palmer, overland travelers to California via the Oregon Trail in the early 1850s were therefore instructed to bring along, per person, "two hundred pounds of flour, thirty pounds of pilot bread, seventy-five pounds of bacon, ten pounds of rice, five pounds of coffee, two pounds of tea, twenty-five pounds of sugar, half a bushel of dried beans, one bushel of dried fruit, two pounds of saleratus [baking soda], ten pounds of salt, half a bushel of corn meal; and it is well to have half a bushel of corn, parched and ground; a small keg of vinegar should also be taken."

Travelers on the Santa Fe Trail and Oregon Trail typically augmented their diet with bison meat—a source of conflict, of course, with Indians, especially when large numbers of bison began to die. The rump, tenderloin, and heart were especially well liked, as was the "marrow gut," a portion of the intestine containing an oily substance resembling bone marrow. The travelers learned to preserve a portion of the kill as jerky, drying it stretched out on the wagon cover as they bounced along the road, trying their best to overlook the dust, insects, and other substances introduced into the meat during the ride. So many bison were killed that a traveler in 1864, Harriet Loughary, recorded that "the bleached bones of buffalo are strewn all along the road"—adding, long before the extermination was finally over, "but not an animal seen. The needless and wanton slaughter of these once numerous animals has almost caused them to be extinct."

The cowboys who arrived early in the Southwest, and whose tastes stamped the Anglo foodways of the region, ate prodigiously. The food was simple but good, for the pay certainly was not: A working cowboy could pretty well count on what came to be known as "three squares," and the best restaurant to be found in many a rural corner was the ranch mess house. One on Charles Goodnight's spread in central Texas was renowned for its cook's liking for chicken, and a reporter for the *Galveston News* recorded in 1886 that the cowboys there ate eggs by the gross and consumed "at least 1000 chickens a year"—and that was just one of many cookhouses scattered across the vast ranch, whose headquarters alone was a village of more than fifty buildings.

What we think of as cowboy cooking was widespread throughout the Anglo Southwest, making full and tedious use of what has been called the Four Bs: beef, beans, biscuits, and bacon. Potatoes, turnips, and corn figured heavily in the region's cuisine, as did pork and sorghum syrup, which rural Southerners were inordinately fond of; when, in Harper Lee's novel *To Kill a Mockingbird*, Scout complains that a young schoolmate is drowning his ham in syrup, the comment is one of class rather than cuisine. Even so, Mark Twain, that Southerner turned Southwesterner turned New Englander, had a lifelong sweet tooth for syrup, and we can forgive his turn to the northeastern woods for the maple trees he found on his land there, putting him in mind of syrup stolen as a child in the perhaps unlikely woods of Missouri. He could remember to the tiniest detail, he wrote, "the taste of maple sap, and when to gather it, and how to arrange the troughs and delivery tubes, and how to boil down the juice, and how to hook the sugar after it is made, and how much better hooked sugar tastes than any that is honestly come by, let bigots say what they will."

The Southwest being notably shy of sap-bearing maples, syrup lovers have

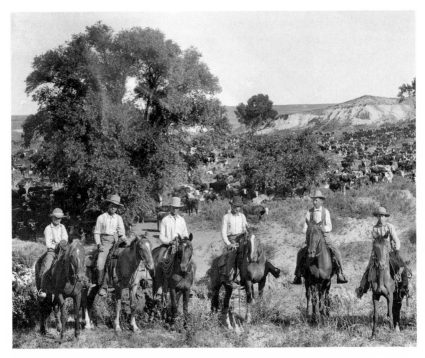

Texas cowboys, 1901. Photograph by William Henry Jackson.

always had to import the stuff. But in much else Anglo Southwesterners soon came to be self-sufficient. About the one thing Anglo Southwesterners did not often make room for on their tables was green vegetables and fresh fruits, which did not hold much esteem in a diet fine-tuned for maximum caloric punch to keep hard-working people working even harder. High fat, carbohydrates, and, for adults, lots of alcohol: The diet was a medical case study in the making.

But once Anglos did arrive in the Southwest in number and began to establish themselves not just as one culture of many but as the dominant culture of the region, the foodways of old became commonplace. If they were from the South, they had the groaning boards of Sunday fried chicken and three vegetables; if from the Northeast, their one-pot meals; if from the Midwest, their milk and cheese. Track their arrival into the region from these different regions and you'll see these dietary differences: Phoenix, where Midwesterners settled in number throughout the early years of the twentieth century, was once ringed by dairy farms, while along the Gila River, in what is aspirationally called Baja Arizona, lay vast chicken farms whose outlines can still be seen today—and some are even in operation.

For all the varied streams of Anglo arrivals into the region, whether from other parts of the United States or from Europe, the Southern influence remained strongest throughout the Southwest, marked from Texas all the way over to Los Angeles. A writer for the New Deal–era Works Progress Administration (WPA) described the foodways of the region in the closing years of the 1930s:

> With an appetite as big as all outdoors, the Southwest eats with gusto. Its taste was early shaped by the spareness of scrub country, the "isolateness" of mountain and desert. The lack of formality that has long characterized its table manners is of pioneer stock, induced by hard living. Of the countless hardships borne in the settlement of this vast region, lack of human companionship was alone insufferable. Eating without formality, then, could satisfy this craving for company better. Fingers in lieu of forks bespoke no impoverishment of living, but more gusto—the appeasement of hidden hunger by the simplest fare, with the variety of all kinds of human companions—stalwart, rogue, and charlatan—to supplement the bare diet afforded. And today the Southwest sets its table with the hospitality of the South, for indeed, many Southerners live there. But this is a hospitality of a gregarious nature—a cordiality that gets in exchange for the giving: the adventurer's yearnings for companionship now deep rooted in the folkways of its tables.

The Southern table dominated. Though never as proverbial as its Southern antecedent, Southwestern hospitality was welcoming and welcome—and often surprisingly so. As late as 1941 a traveler working her way up the fearfully difficult Black Canyon north of Phoenix was delighted to find a kitchen up on a ledge-top settlement that catered to the wildcat miners who worked claims near places like Bumble Bee and Crown King. She reported on the menu she found at the alarmingly named Horse Thief Basin:

> Great, round biscuits—one wondered if they could dispose of one,
>   and ended up by eating three; a bowl of fresh sweet homemade butter;

green onions arranged like a bouquet in a tall spoon holder; cornbread in squares the size and thickness of a cook sized cake of laundry soap, brown and delicious as any that mother used to make; a green earthen mixing bowl of navy beans (the best I ever tasted); a dish of coleslaw; and the piece de resistance was a huge platter of beef. Someone in the vicinity had butchered a yearling. The slices, big as a man's palm, had been pounded, rolled in flour and dropped into heavy iron skillets, deep with lard (this I had seen from my place in the living room). The result was an excellent finished product, a platter of juicy steaks that would have done justice to a Waldorf-Astoria chef. Then there was a veritable Pikes Peak of mashed potatoes, seasoned with butter and pure cream. A bathtub tureen full of steak gravy and a yellow bowl of syrupy dried peaches rounded the menu. Coffee was served once—twice—thrice to several of the huskier miners—and it *was* coffee, rich and black with a delicious aroma and an exhilarating flavor.

Southern again, that food. And there was something at work behind that dominance of Southern cuisine: In the first decades of their dominance in the region, Anglos tended to segregate themselves, settling in communities on the "right side" of the railroad tracks that crossed most towns, establishing covenants and deed restrictions to keep others away. For many years, Anglos parsed the table in terms of our food versus theirs, the cuisine of the Hispanic peoples of the region, who ate bewilderingly hot food cooked in strange ways. Two of the French missionaries who figure in Willa Cather's brilliant 1927 novel *Death Comes for the Archbishop*, a book that describes ethnic tensions in northern New Mexico among Hispanic Catholics and Anglo Protestants in the last half of the nineteenth century, are cases in point. One, Father Vaillant, has most definitely gone native, learning to speak Spanish, ride like a cowboy, and adapt to local customs. "I have almost become a Mexican!" he says. "I have learned to like chili colorado and mutton fat. The Mexicans' foolish ways no longer offend me, their faults are dear to me. I am their man!"

What those "foolish ways" are we cannot say, but in time other non-Hispanic arrivals in the region eventually came around to incorporating elements of Hispanic cuisine into their own daily diets, if in their own way. When I moved to Arizona in 1975, it was not uncommon for an Anglo roadside diner to offer a choice of sandwich bread or a flour tortilla with a meal. The Anglo touch was that the tortilla would be buttered unless specified to be dry. Other efforts were just as, well, syncretic, but not always successful. One cookbook published in Tucson in 1900, for instance, conjured "Spanish sauce" out of "1 ½ pints of water, 1 gill of flour, 1 gill of butter, 2 ounces of lean ham, 3 tablespoonfuls of gelatine, 2 tablespoonfuls of minced onion, 1 tablespoonful of minced carrot, 1 tablespoonful of minced celery, 1 sprig of parsley, 1 bayleaf, 2 whole cloves, a small bit of mace, a generous teaspoonful of salt, ⅓ teaspoonful of pepper." A more venturesome "chili sauce" was made with bell peppers and allspice, hardly the stuff to satisfy a heat-craving diner.

Points are due for effort, one supposes, but it would take a few more decades of living together—or apart together—for a truly Southwestern cuisine to develop. As diets were slowly remade, so too were the agricultural practices of the region, as we will see in the next chapter. But for that change to come, other ingredients were needed, including people from many lands and an entrepreneurial spirit that found that good things could come from blending cowboy cuisine, Southern cooking, and even Midwestern milk with the fiery, smoky, and enchanting tastes they would encounter in the new country.

6. **Extending the Larder**

Walk into the rugged Palos Verdes Hills to the south of Los Angeles, and you gain the rare satisfaction of standing on what is believed to be the fastest-rising bit of real estate on the planet, inching its way ever upward thanks to the force of earthquakes and grinding continental plates. Few places on earth speak so openly of the power of planetary geological forces. As Juan Crespi noted with alarm when he arrived in 1769, no one is a resident of Los Angeles long before experiencing the odd sensation that the earth is little more solid than a bowl of pudding, and everyone knows that it is just a matter of time before the vast San Andreas Fault will awaken, stretch, and shake off layers of buildings, roads, and fields.

And few places boast climates that are at once so mild and so extreme. Los Angeles's famed smog, for instance, is nothing new; when the Spanish explorer Juan Cabrillo dropped anchor off what is now San Pedro in 1542, he called the spot Bahia de los Fumos, or "Bay of Smokes," for the air was dense with the choking exhaust of wildfires and Indian campfires alike. Later promoters of inland communities such as San Bernardino and Rancho Cucamonga promised that buyers would flourish in air free of coastal fog, though the tall mountains that ring the

Los Angeles basin would assure that once the automobile arrived the air would be full of fog of another kind.

Though those promoters and their kin have never liked to talk about it much, Los Angeles sees just about every kind of weather, from moderate to extreme. Thanks to the intersection of mountains, winds, water, and sun, Los Angeles possesses a climate that ecologists rightly classify as "Mediterranean," and for much of the year it rivals the real Mediterranean for clement weather that is not too hot, not too cold, not too wet, not too dry. But because it is perched on the edge of the desert, Los Angeles is subject to intense heat, as well as sandstorms and those patience-testing Santa Ana winds, which seem to create an atmosphere of impending doom. (During their season, as Raymond Chandler wrote in his famous story "Red Wind," "Meek little wives feel the edge of the carving knife and study their husbands' necks. Anything can happen.") Because it lies between a cold ocean and great peaks that block the passage of moisture-laden air, Los Angeles is subject to torrential rains and sometimes paralyzing floods. And because the mountain passes make natural wind tunnels—hence the great fields of electricity-generating windmills at the very place where glaciers once crawled—the Los Angeles basin is subject to tornadoes that would do Kansas proud.

Floods, too. Anglo farmers first came to Southern California in the 1840s. For a decade, struggling to bring grain and produce forth from the earth, they lamented the lack of rain—for coincidentally, the 1840s and '50s were a time of deep drought. In 1861, their prayers for rain were answered with a series of devastating winter storms, the product of the El Niño oscillation. That year, five and a half feet of rain fell, four times as much as normally falls on the region. A newly arrived Californian, William Brewer, wrote to family back east,

> Thousands of farms are entirely under water—cattle starving and drowning. All the roads in the middle of the state are impassable; so all mails are cut off. The telegraph also does not work clear through. In the Sacramento Valley for some distance the tops of the poles are under water. The entire valley was a lake extending from the mountains on one side to the coast range hills on the other. Steamers ran back over the ranches fourteen miles from the river, carrying stock, etc, to the hills. Nearly every house and farm over this immense region is gone. America

has never before seen such desolation by flood as this has been, and seldom has the Old World seen the like.

America *had* seen such flooding before, though 1861 and 1862 were indeed unusual—and for the Southwest devastating, witnessing widespread destruction in places such as Yuma and San Bernardino and wiping out crops throughout the region.

Cyclical shifts in oceanic and air currents explain the Southwest's long record of aridity, punctuated by occasional periods of moderate temperature and even bursts of abnormally cool, wet weather. From time to time, hurricanes blow into the region, as happened in Galveston, Texas, in 1900, killing some eight thousand people in a matter of hours. A great storm front called a *cordonazo* inundated southern Arizona in late September and early October 1983. A tropical storm called Octave, born in the southeastern Pacific, drifted toward Mexico, gathering force as storms will while feeding on accidental antecedents. The previous August and early to mid-September had been unusually moist for the Southwest, and there was plenty of ambient water in the atmosphere already, well ahead of the cyclonic front. Additionally, a mid-latitude cold trough had formed over central Mexico, which pushed that front straight up the warm Gulf of California, where the storm was able to gather still more moisture along the way. And, by happenstance, the surface of the ocean to the west of Mexico's Baja California was at its historic near maximum temperature, which meant that the storm system had plenty of warm water to draw from, and from great distances, keeping its cyclonic rotation alive well north of where such systems usually stall and fade away.

The result: from September 28 to October 3, 1983, a great storm settled over a wedge-shaped area that extended from roughly Las Vegas to below the Colorado Plateau over southern Arizona and New Mexico. Though Octave never touched land, it generated wave after wave of storm fronts, dropping eight inches of rain on Tucson alone in a week, when an average year brings somewhat less than twelve inches. Houses and farmland washed away, bridges and power lines fell, and scores of people were injured or left homeless.

Are Southwesterners prepared for the next *cordonazo* to come? Doubtless not, for the Southwest is growing so fast that in many of the most

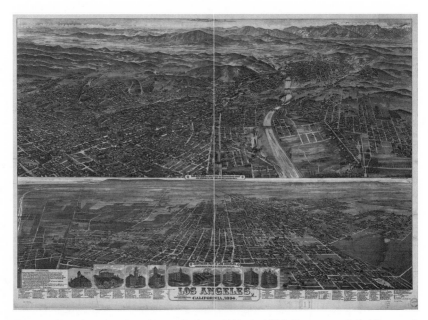

A map of Los Angeles, ringed by agriculture fields, in 1894. Courtesy of the Library of Congress.

storm-sensitive areas, newcomers far outnumber old-timers. If we knew better, those old-timers have long observed, all that water would not be running off the land and running off to other places; if we knew better, there would be no water crisis in the Southwest. But those are a lot of what-ifs, and the old cycle of drought and flood, feast and famine, endures even as a changing climate regime brings hotter average temperatures, which mean increased atmospheric water vapor, the stuff from which storms are made. More storms mean more flooding. More flooding means more soil erosion and the destruction of croplands, estuaries, coastlines. Less productive land means less food. Less food means famine, chaos, and war.

Born on a farm in central Massachusetts in 1849, when newcomers were flooding into the Southwest from around the world, Luther Burbank was the thirteenth of fifteen children, a low position in an already low pecking order. He was spared from farm labor only long enough to complete elementary school then was put to work in the fields and his mother's garden. Young

Santa Rosa Plum Jam

In 1906 the soon-to-be-renowned plant breeder Luther Burbank produced a plum variety that he named the Santa Rosa, after his new California home. The Santa Rosa has since gone on to happy dominion in the world of fruit, grown just about everywhere it can be grown and prized for its compact size and intense sweetness, nicely balanced by a complementary tartness. They also tend to bruise easily when ripe, so they often wind up in jams, jellies, and preserves.

This simple recipe can be adjusted for larger or smaller yields, and chopped skin can be added to the jam for texture. To some tastes, it may want more sugar as well, so adjust to your own liking.

5 pounds plum meat
8 cups sugar
Juice of 2 lemons

Put all ingredients in pot. Bring to a boil, then cover and simmer on very low heat for 20 minutes. Once cool, store the jam in sterilized jars. For added flavor, add lemon peel, basil leaves, cinnamon, or other ingredients—Burbank was an experimenter, and so should we be.

Luther didn't mind, it seems. A bright boy, he read on his own, stacks and stacks of books on botany, agriculture, biology, and other fields, and he loved the hard work of growing food.

We can guess as much because, in 1870, when Burbank was twenty-one, his father died, and he left his son a small but meaningful inheritance. Instead of bolting for the big city, Burbank used the money to buy a place of his own a few miles from the family's farmstead. There, on a fertile seventeen-acre parcel, he continued to experiment with something he had been working on for years: a potato that was capable of withstanding several kinds of pests and viruses, to say nothing of long stretches of bitterly cold weather. That potato proved so successful that Burbank was able to sell the patent rights to it. He did so for only $150, about $2,700 in today's dollars. The fee was tiny, especially considering the fortunes his invention would bring, but again,

Burbank didn't mind. He had been reading all about California, which, he wrote, he pictured as the most perfect farmland on Earth, and he used the money and the proceeds from the sale of his farm in Massachusetts to stake himself to a new home in faraway Santa Rosa.

There Luther Burbank bought a four-acre parcel and began working on new varieties of plants, for by now he had become something more than a self-taught geneticist and evolutionary botanist. He was a full-blown inventor of plants with a talent Gregor Mendel would envy, and there was scarcely a plant grown that he was not interested in improving.

In 1885 Burbank expanded his holdings, buying a fifteen-acre parcel on Gold Ridge, near Sebastopol, about eight miles from his small garden in Santa Rosa, which he had pared down to about an acre as the city began to grow up around him. Using the latter as a kind of showcase and visitor center, he called the Gold Ridge place his "experimental farm," and there he developed thousands of new hybrids, varieties, and crossbred plants, patenting or at least documenting the creation of some eight hundred of them over the decades. Among Burbank's inventions during the half century he spent in the area were the Shasta daisy, the thornless blackberry, and the plum-apricot cross he called the "plumcot." The variety of plants he developed is astonishing, numbering, among others, four kinds each of grapes and pears, ten kinds each of strawberries, apples, and cherries, thirteen kinds of raspberries, sixteen kinds of blackberries, and fully nine dozen kinds of plums and prunes—and those were just the fruits.

During this time, Burbank also began to articulate a kind of aesthetic, or philosophy, of gardening, one that most Americans, whether they know the source or not, follow today. In particular, he encouraged even the hardest-nosed and most practical farmers to reserve at least a little corner for flowers, simply for their enjoyment. "Flowers always make people better, happier, and more helpful; they are sunshine, food and medicine for the soul," he wrote. He also urged gardeners to experiment as he had, keeping good records of what worked and didn't, so that the plants they grew made perfect fits for the places in which they lived.

In all this, Luther Burbank might be considered to be a father of the local-agriculture and locavore movements, even if the plants he introduced to the world spread to every corner of it. He fully defended the global reach of his inventions, too, as when he spoke before an audience in San

Francisco near the very end of his life, saying, "What a joy life is when you have made a close working partnership with Nature, helping her to produce for the benefit of mankind new forms, colors, and perfumes in flowers which were never known before; fruits in form, size, and flavor never before seen on this globe; and grains of enormously increased productiveness, whose fat kernels are filled with more and better nourishment, a veritable storehouse of perfect food—new food for all the world's untold millions for all time to come."

Not all of Burbank's experimental products were runaway successes, even though he enjoyed funding from none other than Andrew Carnegie and, though sometimes accused of being unscientific in his methods, the research support of a number of leading botanists around the world. He developed, for instance, a cross between a petunia and a tobacco plant that seems to have been purely whimsical, one described as a "petunia that had acquired the tobacco habit." He called it the "nicotunia." He also developed a plant that, though a potato, grew on a vine like a tomato. He called it, naturally, the "pomato" but noted that growers were disappointed to learn that it was not actually a hybrid of the two plants. And as for Luther's strawberry-raspberry hybrid, he was disappointed when it did not produce fertile fruit, for he thought the flavors—quite rightly—would be magnificent together.

When Luther Burbank died in 1926, his widow leased most of the experimental farm to a nursery, and over the next thirty-odd years the property slowly went into decline, with Burbank's original plantings fading into the dead and gone. In the late 1970s and early 1980s, the city of Sebastopol began work on restoring Burbank's cottage there, acquiring the building and, eventually, about three acres of the original farm. It is now used as a center for agricultural education.

And as for the potato that Luther Burbank developed way back in the 1870s? Well, another plant geneticist tinkered with his formula a tiny bit to develop a potato with a russet, or dark reddish-brown, skin that sprouted few eyes compared to most other breeds and produced a mealy, dry flesh. Named the Russet Burbank potato in Burbank's honor, the variety quickly spread to farms across the nation and then the world. It and a few closely related cousins, many marketed under the generic term "Idaho potato," are now the most commonly cultivated types of potato in North America, found in every

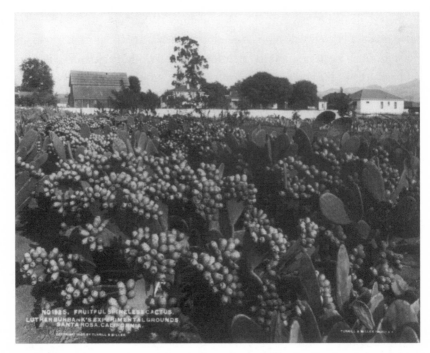

Luther Burbank's experimental farm in Santa Rosa, California, showing various fruiting cacti. Courtesy of the Library of Congress.

grocery store and just about every fast-food restaurant on the continent. If you love french fries, in short, then you owe thanks to Luther Burbank—and if you love flowers, food, and the natural beauty of plants as well.

As an American of predominantly Irish and Swedish ancestry, I harbor mixed feelings about the potato, the genius of Luther Burbank notwithstanding. It is delicious, of course, and essential, but also instrumental in the cruel diaspora that nearly emptied the mother country of its people and sent kin off to America, where, in the words of the lyricist Phillip Chevron, we would evermore "celebrate the land that made us refugees."

The potato was first cultivated in the Bolivian highlands, the toxins of the Solanum genus bred out by generations of agricultural experimentation, and by the time the Europeans arrived, its production extended far northward into the highlands of Mexico. The potato was soon introduced to Spain. At the same time, it came into English hands, and it was then, in a roundabout caps —

ly—

stay—

way, introduced to the colony of Virginia, where it flourished so much in the highlands that it came to be known as the "Virginia potato." It spread into the cuisine of the South from that source, even as it became common in numerous European cuisines, particularly in what Simon Winder has happily called the nonexistent but very real polylingual land of Danubia.

The potato thus came into the Southwest from many directions: from missionaries stationed at Spanish posts in Texas and California, by way of Southern cooking, in the farming regimes of immigrants from Central and Eastern Europe, and by Mormon farmers who came into the region from the north and east, carrying their counting rhyme "one potato, two potato, three potato, four" with them.

In California and Arizona potatoes were again largely associated with Mormon farmers. In New Mexico they grew in Spanish and Anglo fields alike, and there a young man named Deak Parsons encountered them, ruefully remembering that he lost the state's spelling bee in 1914 by leaving the "e" out of their name. Parsons, who lived his happiest years in Fort Sumner, where Billy the Kid met his end, would gain fame as the bombardier of the *Enola Gay*, which carried the atomic bomb, field-tested not far from Parsons's childhood home, to Hiroshima, Japan.

Potatoes are an economically important crop in parts of Texas, especially the northern Panhandle and lower Rio Grande valley, but they are less extensively planted even there than most other crops, including sunflowers and grapefruit. This may reflect the fact that American potato consumption has fallen from the 200 or so pounds eaten per capita in 1900 to the 120-odd pounds we eat today. Even so, as vegetables go—even though the potato is not, in strictest terms, a vegetable—it occupies pride of place on the American table, particularly when accompanied by condiments made from a close runner-up, the tomato.

Solanum lycopersicum, which is Latin for "sunbeam wolf peach," or earlier, *Lycopersicon esculentum*, which is Latin for "succulent wolf peach," briefly confounded the Spanish who first encountered it in the Caribbean, for, they whispered of the strange-tasting plant, it was a natural aphrodisiac. Despite its reputation, or perhaps surreptitiously because of it, it found its way into mission gardens throughout the Southwest. Championed by none other than Thomas Jefferson, it also found its way into Southern cuisine, and from those two sources, Virginian and Spanish, it became a staple

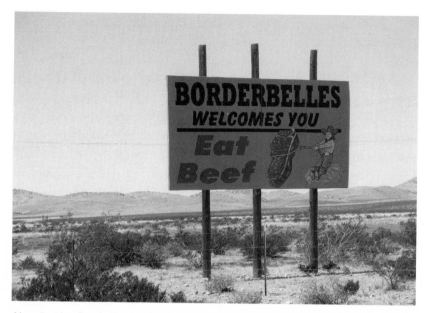

Abundant beef underlies much of the Southwest's exported cuisine.

of Southwestern cooking, grown and consumed everywhere in the region and centrally important to the region's cuisine. Tomatoes are versatile things, whether you consider them a vegetable or a fruit, and there are abundant ways to prepare them. In the form of ketchup, we can put them on our french fries. We can chop them up raw and put them on our tacos in the form of salsa cruda, that wonderful mix of tomatoes, peppers, maybe a cucumber, a sprig of cilantro, and a scallion or two, and maybe some tomatillo, or we can cook them with peppers and make taco sauce of them that way. Just about any way of preparing them does honor to a plant whose genetic sequence, decoded in part at the University of Arizona in 2012, contains some thirty-five thousand parts—about seven thousand more than that of human beings.

The agriculture of New Mexico, California, and eastern Texas has always been richer than that of Arizona, generally speaking. Apart from obvious meteorological and ecological factors, there is good historical reason for this difference: Where the Spanish were able to settle in those richer areas within the course of a few years, in Arizona it took more than a century before significant portions of the countryside could be pacified, thanks to the fierce resistance of the Apaches along the northern frontier of New Spain.

The missions along the lower Rio Grande of New Mexico, particularly Socorro and El Paso, were renowned for their agricultural richness, thanks to a priest named Fray Garcia de San Francisco. Arriving on the Rio Grande in 1659, the good brother was an avid botanist and gardener with a spectacularly green thumb. Many of his seeds and cuttings were brought to other settlements in New Mexico and Texas, making him a kind of Southwestern antecedent to Johnny Appleseed.

Agriculture also attracted everyone who came to Southern California, it seemed, Spanish or otherwise. For example, Joseph Chapman—no known relation to John Chapman, the aforementioned Johnny Appleseed—who is known to local history as "Pirate Joe," arrived in California in 1818 as a crewmember on one of the last pirate ships to ply its coast. Captured by the Spanish, he was sent to Los Angeles with instructions to teach the Indians there how to build a church. He had learned carpentry skills along the way, as well as some medical tricks, and he made himself invaluable around San Gabriel. When his duty to the mission was finished, he launched a commercial winegrowing enterprise and grew numerous other crops in the San Gabriel area as well. In 1839 he moved his enterprises to Santa Barbara, where he died a decade later.

Thomas Starr King, a farmer and early booster of its agriculture, advertised California's bounty in an address of 1862:

> California is sketched out by the Almighty as a vast canvas, such as no tribe of men ever received, for the genius and fidelity of colonists to fill with beauty. One of our own citizens has recently indulged an artist's dream of what the State might look like a hundred years hence. He sees in vision 'long ribbons of fields stretching to Fort Tejon'—each field a different color—green grapes, brown furrows, emerald vines, fringing hedges; grains growing, cream-colored grains, grains aureate and russet; houses dotted along like violets in flower-beds; houses reaching forth like mosses in the crystal brook; houses clumped, houses grouped, hamlets modest, hamlets blooming and luxuriant like gorgeous creepers; villages with spires, towns with burnished domes goldened by the sun, and silvered by

the moon; cities with minarets, cities with columns, cities with tall needle chimneys pouring up to God the frankincense of labor; terraced foot-hills laughing with generous villas, sloping forelands alive with herds; swelling mounds nestling with vines, oval knolls crowned with festoons of fruit blossoms, breathing sweet perfume to the sky; mountain gorges rolling out metals, mountain peaks staring at opposite peaks from bold-faced palaces, mountain rivulets murmuring to trellised rose-hidden cottages, mountain vales creeping away to love God in dreamy repose.

Those who followed King extended that exalted vision. At the missions of California, Junípero Serra and other clerics had introduced sweet oranges, lemons, and limes to the missions of Southern California, with the first sizable orange grove established at Mission San Gabriel in 1804. William Wolfskill, a German immigrant, arrived in Los Angeles in 1831 and planted a small grove from seeds that he acquired at the mission, the basis for a modest citrus empire that would eventually grow to more than seventy acres and give birth to the modern Southern California citrus industry.

But we need to backtrack. Introduced by Christopher Columbus on his second voyage, oranges, lemons, and other citrus fruit trees were widely planted in the Southwest well before Anglo settlers arrived. It is a curiosity that they first arrived in what is now Arizona, brought by the great Jesuit missionary Eusebio Francisco Kino to the missions he established along the Río Sonora and the Santa Cruz. In a report of 1707 to royal officials, he wrote of the mission gardens, "There are many Castilian fruit trees such as fig trees, quinces, oranges, pomegranates, peaches, apricots, pear-trees, apples, mulberries, pecans, prickly pears, etc., with all sorts of garden stuff."

Oranges would not arrive in California for another half century, but when they did, at San Diego in 1769, they were widely planted in orchards far more extensive than the home stands of Arizona. When the British explorer George Vancouver visited the mission at San Buenaventura in what is now Ventura, California, in 1793, he recorded the cultivation of a pleasing variety of fruits: "apples, pears, plumbs, figs, oranges, grapes, peaches, and pomegranates, together with the plantain, banana, cocoa nut, sugar cane, indigo." He also noted the presence of "great quantities of the Indian fig, or prickly pear; but whether cultivated for its fruit only or for the cochineal I was not able to make myself thoroughly acquainted."

Even so, it was not until the 1880s, after the introduction of industrial-scale agriculture to now-American California, that oranges and lemons were grown in large commercial quantities, recorded at fifteen million boxes of fruit annually in the first decade of the twentieth century. Most of these commercial orchards radiated outward from the old Spanish mission of San Gabriel, just north and east of Los Angeles, the descendants of the four hundred or so orange trees the missionaries planted there; many of them were still active until finally overwhelmed by the urbanization and suburbanization of Southern California in the postwar period, when citrus groves moved eastward into the Imperial and Colorado River valleys, with the last of the original mission trees dying in San Bernardino in 1961.

Nearby, in the religious community of Riverside, the newly introduced navel orange was first planted in 1873. Five years later some seventeen thousand orange trees filled the air with the heady scent of blossoms, just in time for the completion of the southern route of the transcontinental railway in 1876. The most prominent orange in the early years was the Valencia, and even after the arrival of the navel orange from Brazil, it remained popular enough that the California Fruit Growers Exchange, established in 1902 and reorganized half a century later as Sunkist, devoted much of its efforts to promoting Valencia production.

In 1877 the first of countless shipments of California oranges went east, at first only to St. Louis, then onward to New York. After the refrigerated boxcar was introduced in 1889, they traveled even farther, with five carloads shipped all the way to London, a voyage lasting nearly a month on railcar and then steamship. So great was demand for California oranges that by the 1920s fifty thousand railroad carloads were being shipped east each year and thirty years later almost 250,000 acres of land in Los Angeles county were devoted to citrus farming.

In Texas, with its generally dryer but warm climate, growers paid note to California's success. By the late 1880s small orange groves were flourishing around Houston, though periodic freezes kept a large-scale industry from developing elsewhere in the state except in the lower Rio Grande Valley. New Mexico, similarly, was too high in elevation and too cold to sustain citrus, leaving it to California and Arizona to lead the region in production. It would take some years for the orange juice industry to develop in California and elsewhere in the Southwest; then and now, while it sometimes runs second to the offshoot industry in Florida, it is an important plank in the region's agriculture.

My father, who lived in Pasadena as a boy, remembers the smell of oranges everywhere he went in springtime in Southern California. Citrus groves have long since given way to strip malls and freeways, but if you have ever smelled an orange tree in blossom, you know how tragic this is at heart—how sad that the small desert city of Pomona, named after the Roman goddess of fruit, has become just another place without much in the way of agriculture to commend it, how sad that some of the most productive farmland in the world, as the classicist and farmer Victor Davis Hanson has documented in his book *Fields without Dreams*, should now lie under building foundations and parking lots.

Traveling across the desert in 1861, Mark Twain stopped at a stagecoach station and asked for a cup of coffee. The stationmaster was speechless by way of reply. Finally he sputtered, "*Coffee!* Well, if that don't go clean ahead of me, I'm damned!" About the best the station could do was rancid bacon, stale bread, some vinegar that had gone off even by the standards of vinegar, and slumgullion, a blend of tea and what Twain called "dish-rag and sand." Not long before, Sir Richard Burton, the discoverer of the Nile's source, had made a similar trek in the American desert, and he wrote that the bacon was "rusty" and the coffee boiled and boiled again "till every noxious principle was duly extracted from it," while the bread was made of alkali and sour milk that combined to make a brew that "communicates to the food a green-yellow tinge, and suggests many of the properties of poison."

In that light, an antelope steak "cut off a corpse suspended for the benefit of flies outside," as Burton described it, constituted something of a feast. It would be just a few years, though, before the completion of the transcontinental railroad would essentially put an end to the stagecoach as a primary means of transport across the Southwest, and with that technological leap came a thoroughgoing change in the production of food in the region. Whereas in 1800 it took six weeks for a New Yorker to travel to the banks of the Mississippi River, at the end of the nineteenth century it took that many days to cross the whole continent to San Francisco. The railroad brought seafood, too: By the 1880s, live oysters from the Chesapeake Bay were on sale in Santa Fe, transported across the country in large wooden barrels that were packed first with oysters, then with shaved ice, then with cornmeal, and so on in layers until the barrel was filled. As a train crossed the country, it put in at icehouses to replenish the ice. "By the time the live oysters arrived in Santa Fe," relates chef and food historian Holly Arnold Kinney, "they were more plump and delicious than when they were pulled out of the bay."

The railroad changed everything. Not long after the golden spike was

Huevos Rancheros

The Fred Harvey Company did more than a single enterprise's share to promote the exchange of regional foods while keeping customers in its railroad hotels and restaurants happy. This recipe, from the often-reprinted *Santa Fe Super Chief Cook Book*, is credited to a German-born chef named Konrad Allgeier, who trained in Zurich before heading the kitchen at the renowned La Fonda of Santa Fe. That may explain the fondness for butter in this recipe, which, for all that, produces tasty and reasonably authentic results.

1 cup pinto beans
1 tablespoon red chili powder
¼ cup water
4 tablespoons minced onion
½ to 1 teaspoon finely minced green chili pepper
2 tablespoons butter
2 eggs
1 teaspoon butter

Wash beans, cover with cold water, and let soak overnight. In the morning, heat to boiling, reduce heat and let simmer, covered, until beans are tender: 3 or 4 hours. Cool. Add red chili powder, which may be obtained from a Mexican grocery store, to the cold water and let soak one hour. Sauté onion and very finely minced green chili pepper in butter very slowly until tender but not browned. Add beans, which have been broken up coarsely with a fork and heat through. Add ¼ to ½ cup hot water if beans are too dry. Transfer heated beans to a well-buttered shirred egg dish or individual casserole. Make two depressions in top of beans using back of tablespoon, and drop an egg in each depression. Pour 2 tablespoons soaked red chili powder over the top and dot top of eggs with butter. Bake in a moderate oven (350° F), 20 to 25 minutes or until eggs are set sufficiently. Yield: one serving.

sunk in Utah, a traveler and restaurateur who had endured many a bad meal on the road divined that he could use speed of transport to his advantage. Fred Harvey had worked his way up the line from busboy to owner, and he knew his finnan haddie and his cheese soup. His idea was simple: At stops across the prairie into the Southwest on the route of the Atchison, Topeka, and Santa Fe, he would build travelers' inns serving fresh food in wondrous quantities. As a refinement of the idea, he soon hit on the notion that this fresh food would be served by young women whom he called "Harvey Girls." Dozens of his Harvey Houses sprang up along and near railroad lines throughout the Southwest, and it is no accident that some of the finest hotels in the region today are also Harvey creations or allies with fine restaurants attached, including La Fonda in Santa Fe and the Turquoise Room of La Posada in Winslow, Arizona.

Fred Harvey favored sturdy food to fit his taste, educated but rooted in the working-class Liverpool from which he had immigrated. He bought beef by the stockyard—more than twelve hundred pounds a week early on—and daringly served it less than shoe-leather well done, educating Southwestern palates himself. Moreover, along with the blue point oysters, halibut, and potatoes au gratin, Harvey served local dishes, for one of his fundamental rules of doing business was, "Never take yourself too damn seriously," and one of the sure signs of doing so was being slavish to an East Coast culinary regime. A Harvey House chef in Las Vegas, New Mexico, was renowned up and down the line for his albondigas soup, to which he added a few exotic ingredients such as butter and marjoram. Harvey liked his codfish balls and his sautéed bullfrogs, but he may have been the first Anglo restaurateur in the nation to serve guacamole to Anglo guests. A collection of his recipes made certain cultural adjustments, to be sure; as one for "chili sauce" put it, "The foregoing is a Mexican dish, but the average American prefers a some-what milder sauce, which can be produced by one quart or more of tomatoes instead of water."

Harvey House cookbooks made room for other ethnic cuisines as well, serving up Hungarian goulash and German potato salad, French pancakes and even something approximating spaghetti. The same was true of other purveyors of food for a mass audience of travelers, forerunners of the fast food restaurants that we will visit in a later chapter. When in 1911 Harry Luby founded the chain of restaurants that would bear his name, his menu allowed for enchiladas and guacamole; his successors would even add a Texas-style chop suey to the mix. But for the most part Luby's stuck to a solidly Southern repertoire heavy on baked ham, chicken potpie, three vegetables, and gelatin. As a very young child living in El Paso, I eagerly awaited visits to Luby's and its triple threat of starches—mashed potatoes, french fries, and macaroni and cheese—that are resolutely unadventurous, to be sure, but are the very definition of comfort food. It goes without saying that Jell-O was the dessert of choice.

By the time Luby began to build his empire, Southwestern agriculture was fully industrialized, and nearly any ingredient that a chef could have wanted was readily available in season. Texas and California pioneered large-scale farms growing industrial crops—at first cotton, then other commodities such as wheat and raisins. Small farms of fewer than 160 acres, operated by individuals rather than cooperatives or corporations, abounded until the modern era. Some of these were barely at subsistence level; as the *Handbook of Texas* notes, a 120-acre farm might see a hundred of those acres used for livestock grazing, mostly pigs and cows, while twelve acres would be used to raise corn, mostly for feed, and another two or three acres would be used to raise cotton to bring in a little cash. The rest of the acreage, a postage stamp by comparison, would house a cane field, a garden, and a few beds of tobacco, altogether keeping body and soul together but seldom making much of a fortune for anyone involved.

Still, the farm economy was diverse and prolific. In Texas American settlers from the South introduced the honeybee; though the Spanish had cultivated a great many crops there, introducing, for example, barley and oats in the 1730s, cabbage and lettuce in the 1760s, and beets and carrots in the 1830s, honey was apparently not one of them. Honeybees arrived in Texas in the 1830s, and from there they spread to other parts of the Southwest, joining hives brought in elsewhere by more apiculturally inclined friars and missionaries. On that note, the first olive grove in Southern California was established at the San Fernando mission. When the Franciscans abandoned the mission, olive growing was almost forgotten in the area until, in the late 1890s, a businessman named Robert Widney established a commercial olive orchard near Sylmar, using mostly Chinese workers. His farm, at one time the largest olive grove in the world, remained in operation until the 1960s.

Fertile and seemingly without end, the interior valleys of California saw vast production of just about every crop under the sun, just as Thomas Starr King had promised that it would. Among other crops, California was long a world leader in the production of apples, for instance, while grains, vegetables of all kinds, nuts, grapes, fruits, tomatoes, avocados—well, as with the black soil of Virginia, it seemed that anything that was planted in the California earth would spring up healthy and endless.

Arizona, more arid and austere, was also more challenging. In some things it excelled, though. The North African date palm, for instance, was introduced there in the nineteenth century. Earlier, North African date palm trees were grown in small numbers in missions in Baja California and on the California coast, but the climate was not amenable to large-scale production. That of the Lechuguilla Desert in the blazingly hot desert country between Yuma and Gila Bend was—and today a little town called Dateland stands to commemorate that industry—its most welcome manifestation, served courtesy of a roadside diner that serves icy date milkshakes to thirsty travelers. There are plenty of good uses to put dates to apart from milkshakes, though, for they are the sweetest of all generally available fruits and contain more potassium than bananas, with a much lower calorie count. Given the looming need for highly productive foods of all kinds, dates—which also grow abundantly in the Coachella Valley of Southern California—may very well be a fruit in need of discovery and rediscovery.

Up until World War II, about a quarter of all Texans worked on farms. That number steadily fell after the war, a combination of the growth of the industrial and then service economies and the mechanization of agriculture as food production became more and more corporate and less and less the province of individual farmers. The same pattern has held throughout the Southwest. There have been holdouts, of course. The so-called Little Lander movement flourished in California after 1913, when it was founded by a man named William Smythe, who spread a doctrine that a farm could grow enough to sustain a family on just one or two acres. His utopian movement was focused on the area around Tujunga, located next door to the more industrially oriented Burbank—named not for Luther but David, a dentist turned sheep baron and real estate magnate. Smythe attracted a few adherents elsewhere in Southern California, but it has only been recently that his theory has been revived, with many smallholder farms springing up throughout Southern California as part of a new back-to-the-land movement, as if to say that, indeed, everything old is new again.

Water flows indifferently east or west, says the Chinese philosopher Mencius. It does not flow indifferently up or down.

In the arid Southwest, Mencius's axiom has a corollary: Indifferent or not, water can be made to flow uphill toward money. In the nineteenth and twentieth centuries, money brought pharaonic civil-engineering programs like the Central Arizona Project and the All-American Canal to the desert; money brought the water that has made boomtowns of Phoenix and Las Vegas, among the fastest-growing metropolises in the United States throughout the postwar era, when air conditioning and improved communication and transportation networks made urban life in the desert seem not just possible but even attractive.

Both water and money in the region were once broadly distributed among farms, ranches, mines, and towns. In the postwar era, both were increasingly concentrated in the cities of the West, lending the decades-long struggle over water rights a new dimension: the metropolis versus the countryside. Nowhere has this division been more acutely seen than in Southern California, a lush land claimed from the Mojave Desert through the work of boosters like Joseph B. Lippincott, a developer who lobbied Theodore Roosevelt to create the National Reclamation Act, and Frederick Eaton, a onetime farmer in Owens Valley, two hundred miles north of Los Angeles, who moved to the growing city and became a booster and politician.

Eaton was not especially adept at either farming or politics, but he had a clear view of the future. Southern California, he argued, could not grow without a steady supply of water. That water was to be found in Owens Valley, he said, in quantities "adequate for any requirement Los Angeles may ever have." Water czar William Mulholland concurred, and in 1903 he sent Eaton north to Owens Valley to buy up vacant properties in order to acquire water rights and secure territory for a great gravity canal. Ten years later, Owens Valley water was spilling down the new Los Angeles Aqueduct to the city.

Yet Owens Valley was not enough "for any requirement Los Angeles may ever have." In 1941 the aqueduct was extended to Mono Lake. Its water fueled Los Angeles's growth for a while, but it, too, was not enough, and Los Angeles sued its neighbors for ever-greater shares of the Colorado River. That water was not forthcoming, Arizona and New Mexico having successfully combined to keep 2.8 million acre-feet of water out of the Southland's reach.

In recent years the thirsty metropolis has turned its attention closer to home, buying up the farmlands of central California for water. Phoenix has been doing the same with the farms and ranches of the Arizona desert, and some Texas municipalities have been following suit in the wake of uncertainty about water supply in the last few drought-ridden years. The consequent decline of agriculture, which uses 80 percent of the available water throughout the region, had enabled Southern California, Phoenix, Austin, San Antonio, and other cities to grow by scarcely imaginable leaps, even as agricultural fields are put out of production, an economic change made possible only by the development of a global network that allows consumers in the region to buy their winter produce from places such as Australia and Chile instead of the winter fields of the Central Valley and the lower Colorado River. By 2050, state planners project, California's population will reach more than fifty million. If present trends of growth continue, by 2090 the number could be three hundred million.

Without agriculture, the state has sufficient water to fuel such growth; California's is a mere problem of trading fresh lettuce and avocados for an endless strip mall stretching from Blythe to Seal Beach, from Eureka to El Centro. A similar pattern holds for the rest of the arid Southwest. Futurists predict that Arizona, now with somewhat less than seven million residents, can grow to a population of twenty-five million if agricultural water can be reallocated to municipal use. Cities like El Paso and Albuquerque, Sierra Vista and Bakersfield are booming, and as what Wallace Stegner called the "oasis civilization" of the West becomes increasingly urbanized—and Arizona's population, for one, is more urban than New York's—the battle over water rights will increasingly favor the cities, where political power resides.

When Anglo farmers first arrived in the Gila River valley of central Arizona, for example, they dammed the stream and its tributaries to make reservoirs. The water stopped flowing to Indian villages, which prompted a group of Akimel O'odham to set out for Washington to seek an audience with President Ulysses S. Grant. It was some weeks before they were able to call on the president, to whom a delegate said, "Until the past few years we have always had plenty of water to irrigate our farms and never knew what want was. We always had grain stored up for a full year's supply. We were happy and contented. Since the white man came and built the big canals and ditches, we have no water for crops. The government refuses to give us food and we do not ask for it. We can only ask for water, for we prefer to earn our own living if we can."

Mindful, perhaps, of the fact that Indians were not then citizens and therefore could not vote, Grant suggested that they move to Oklahoma. The Akimel O'odham decided to stay in their homeland. Whereas they had been selling fields of wheat to the US government during the Civil War, by 1880 the government was giving them 225,000 pounds of wheat each year. By 1887 the diversion dams upriver had turned nearly the entire river away from its course, and only a quarter of their once-extensive fields were arable. George Webb, who died in 1965, recounted that transformation, recalling a place that the Akimel O'odham called New York Thicket because the cottonwoods were as tall as skyscrapers:

> The green of those Pima fields spread along the river for many miles in the old days when there was plenty of water.
> Now the river is an empty bed full of sand.
> Now you can stand in that same place and see the wind tearing pieces of bark off the cottonwood trees along the dry ditches.

Agriculture is declining throughout the arid regions of the world, largely because irrigation exacts an unsustainable level of environmental damage. In Australia, Central Asia, and the Near East, as well as in North America, once-productive desert fields lie idle, covered in a shield of desert salts that irrigation water has left behind. "In the 1990s," wrote environmental journalist Russell Clemings in that transitional decade, "we may finally understand that what we have done to our deserts in the quest for ever-greater quantities of food carries a hidden cost as well. Irrigation can poison the land and water, it can cripple birds and make fish toxic, and worst of all, its undeniable benefits may prove to be fleeting."

In that regard, it is a small irony that almonds, having recently been dubbed a wonder food of substantial nutritional benefit to figure-conscious diners everywhere, have also become something of a scapegoat for California's latest, and undeniably serious, water crisis. The product of a drought that shows every sign of equaling the one that helped bring about the end of the great Ancestral Puebloan cities of the Southwest, this crisis has forced a debate about just where California's priorities lie: in the fields or on the freeways. California grows 80 percent of the world's almond crop, valued at a little more than $4.3 billion. Botanically not a nut but a seed, the almond is a thirsty thing, and California growers have long been accustomed to giving it groundwater to drink, groundwater whose supplies have been shrinking quickly enough to occasion lawsuits and rationing schemes. Remarks economist David Zetland, "The people of the state of California are more or less destroying themselves in order to give cheap almonds to the world. . . . The problem is that California, because of its failed institutions for managing water, is allowing these almonds to come on market at $3–$4 a pound wholesale, when the price would be tripled if California was managing its water sustainably and farmers faced the real cost of water."

Will the Southwest be farmland, or will it be metropolis? In that question, which defines the current debate, there is no allowance for the arid region as it is—as a place in need of care as all places are, one that should exist on its own terms. "Because we're humans, it's logical to look at nature for food, for cures," remarked the late naturalist Ann Zwinger. "But we must also recognize that there are less easily identifiable values that lie in another dimension, a worth that is more, much more, than what is obvious." The Southwest's intangible worth is obvious to many of us who live here, but even that recognition will likely not soon resolve the fierce water wars that are raging within its austere confines, wars that will in turn decide the future of food in the Southwest.

7. **African Americans**

When, in 1781, the Spanish crown first established a settlement in what is now Los Angeles and what was then the province of Alta California, twenty-six of the forty-four original colonists were of African descent. Most were mulatos from the western coastal province of Sinaloa, a region with long connections to California. A few years later, an offshoot rancho was established in the San Fernando Valley, its owner another African named Francisco Reyes. And just a few years after that, in 1801, an African Mexican child was born at the San Gabriel Mission, a few miles southeast of present-day Pasadena. His name was Pio de Jesús Pico, and over his long life—he died in 1894—he would serve, among other things, as the last Mexican governor of California.

When Pio was a young man, he would have met a newcomer neighbor, another Mexican of African descent named María Rita Valdez de Villa, who built an adobe home on what is now Sunset Boulevard. Granted a 4,500-acre ranch by the Spanish viceroy of New Spain just before Mexico won its independence, Valdez established a thriving business as a cattle rancher. After thirty years of such work, she retired, selling the property to developers who in turn sold it off for small farmsteads, dotting the low hills with wheat and bean fields, walnut groves, and

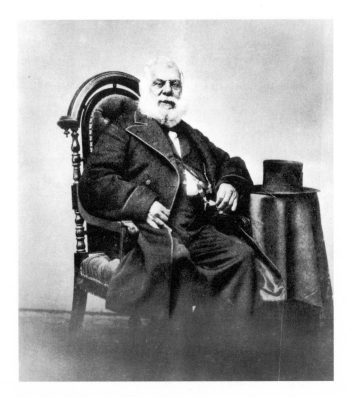

Pio de Jesús Pico, the African Mexican pioneer who served as Mexico's last governor of Alta California. Courtesy of California State Parks.

beehives. This area bore several names, including Santa Maria and Villa Ranch, to honor the original owner. Eventually a developer who had moved from Beverly Farms, Massachusetts, bought most of the former ranch, calling it at first Beverly and then, as of 1907, Beverly Hills.

The first African American in the Southwest, allowing for broad interpretation of at least a couple of those terms, was Estevánico, the "Moor" we met earlier. In her 2014 novel *The Moor's Account*, Laila Lalami gives him the resonant name Mustafa ibn Muhammad ibn Abdussalam al-Zamori and establishes him as a rival storyteller to Alvar Nuñez Cabeza de Vaca—for if history belongs to the victor, as it is said, then it also belongs to the one most likely to enjoy the favor of an influential audience, and a slave would probably not fill that role. Lalami did not have to imagine the fact of Estevánico's sad end, which occurred after the governor of the province of Nueva Galicia, Francisco Vásquez de Coronado, sent him and a priest named Marcos de Niza to the northern frontier of New Spain with orders to locate the cities of gold that Cabeza de Vaca had let slip existed somewhere off over the horizon. De Niza returned to Mexico, saying that he had found those cities but that Estevánico had run afoul of Zuni men who, perhaps jealous that the Moor had inserted himself into local politics and local hammocks alike, killed him.

Other Africans followed Estevánico into New Mexico during the colonial era. One, a Congolese named José Antonio, arrived in El Paso in 1752 and made his way to Santa Fe, where he married an Apache woman known to history only as Marcela. In the colonial capital he found descendants of other mixed marriages, among them the grandchildren of Sebastián Rodriguez Brito, an Angolan who had taken part in the expedition organized by Governor Don Diego de Vargas in 1692 to retake the colony after a revolt by Pueblo Indians. For his services Brito was awarded land in the territory and was one of the wealthiest residents of Santa Fe in the early eighteenth century. Other *genízaros*, or people of mixed race, settled in the northern New Mexico village of Las Trampas in the 1750s, their bloodline containing not just African ancestors but also indigenous peoples from Tlaxcala who had allied with Hernán Cortés in the conquest of Aztec Mexico.

Africans, in short, have been a presence in the Southwest since the early days of the European entradas, and if their contributions always seem to be mentioned as an afterthought, they have surely shaped the history, culture, and cuisine of the region.

Most African Americans entered the region as enslaved people, of course, some illegally held in Texas and elsewhere in the Southwest when they were part of Mexico, in which slavery had been outlawed. That was one of the precipitating factors of the Texas Revolution, which established slavery as a lawful and thriving activity in the newly independent republic. Following the Civil War and emancipation, African Americans became a significant part of the population of Texas, about six hundred thousand in 1900 and nearly a million by the end of World War II. Until the 1940s their numbers were very small elsewhere in the region, though they made their presence known in numerous ways. Many of the cowboys who worked the southwestern ranges

130

were African Americans, for instance, as were the soldiers who bore the nickname, bestowed by Native Americans, of "buffalo soldiers." Among the first African Americans to settle in Tucson were Henry Merchant, who had been a cowboy and cook who briefly ran a restaurant in town, and Joe Mitchell, who raised chickens while operating one of downtown's busiest barbershops.

Robert Owens bought his freedom from slavery on a Texas cotton farm and made for California, arriving in Los Angeles at about the same time as Mitchell and Merchant did in Tucson in 1853. Owens steadily built a fortune in real estate by acquiring less-desirable portions of land that became highly wanted once the valleys and hills began to fill with houses. Many of his early clients were other African Americans, who founded businesses and restaurants. The African American population of Los Angeles grew steadily throughout the late nineteenth and early twentieth centuries until, by 1930, it had the largest population of black residents on the West Coast, numbering about twenty thousand.

African American neighborhoods formed near downtown Los Angeles at places like Sugar Hill in the West Adams district, though such places were hemmed in by color lines that were not widely crossed until the 1940s, when an influx of black workers recruited from the South for wartime industries increased the African American population more than tenfold. The population overall jumped in California during that time, which went from about seven million residents in 1940 to nine and a half million in 1945, with African Americans disproportionate in the migration: the entire African American population west of the Mississippi was about 170,000 in 1940, but 625,000 in 1945.

Those migrants of the nineteenth and twentieth centuries brought Southern food traditions with them, the food of the rural backwaters, places in which, as chef Dora Charles rightly puts it, "country people . . . had to make do with what was at hand, what they could grow or trade or preserve." Their characteristic dishes were things such as hoppin' John, smothered squirrel, hush puppies, collard greens, pigs' feet, ham hocks, fatback, and fried chicken. Peas, greens, field beans, sweet potatoes, okra, bread and syrup—these were the common foods of rural workers white and black in the South and parts of the Southwest well into our own era, before processed foods took their place. Rupert Vance noted in his 1932 book *Human Geography of the South* that "the vast majority of Negroes and many more white people than commonly realized live the year around on such a diet," and he was of course right; for many African Americans, and many poor whites, for that matter, more expensive options such as pork roast or beef were rare and exotic treats, which gives specific gravity to Eldridge Cleaver's remark in his 1968 memoir *Soul on Ice*, "The people in the ghetto want steaks. Beef steaks. I wish I had the power to see to it that the bourgeoisie really did have to make it on soul food."

Soul food was thus where it was at. Consider okra, a vegetable that for a very long time would never dare show itself on a Southern table meant to serve white company, to say nothing of restaurants. A member of the mallow family, closely related to cotton, and the only one eaten as a vegetable, okra (*Hibiscus esculentus*) was first cultivated in its native Horn of Africa but was widely adopted elsewhere in Africa. In the Bantu-speaking western lands that were the chief sources for the transatlantic slave trade, okra was called *ki ngombo*, the origin of the word "gumbo." Africans took the plant with them into captivity, and it enters the historical record in the American South in the 1680s. Grown in garden plots and small farms, it became a staple of the slave diet, the food of poor people, until it was reclaimed, along with greens and beans and other infra dig foods, as a point of pride in the lexicon of soul food. If there is *a* soul food, it might well be okra, which is now featured on smart menus around the country.

In that respect, okra is much like chicken and waffles, a current hit in hipster restaurants throughout the nation. Many a food writer has claimed that the dish originated in Harlem in restaurants catering to jazz musicians, who tended to finish their workday long after dinner had been served and before breakfast was on the table; the middle-ground concoction of chicken and waffles, by that account, embraced both meals. However, well before the Civil War, Virginians were eating just such a meal, the "Virginia breakfast," featuring fried or baked meats including chicken with hot bread or pancakes. Black cooks, of course, prepared these meals, and it is through them that the dish has been translated over the decades into what is increasingly mainstream culture today.

As meats go, chicken is cheap—and thus a common fixture of the diets of poor people around the world. The same thing is true with corn, which many an African would have eaten well before being pressed into service in the New World, planted in the 1500s first around slave ports and then everywhere in the continent, along with peanuts, chiles, sweet potatoes, and other American crops. In the Columbian exchange of plants, Africa contributed a few to the Americas in turn, one of them being sorghum, the source of the syrup that figures prominently in the traditional southern diet as well.

Cornbread in all its forms is a sine qua non of that diet, perhaps most happily in the African American comfort food called the hush puppy—good for quieting dogs, to be sure, but also just about any sort of existential malaise that life can throw at a person.

One variant on cornbread has mostly associated with the Mississippi Delta for generations, having migrated there from the Southwest: the tamale. On quick inspection, it is clear that this tamale is that thing of Mesoamerican origin that Cortés encountered soon after arriving in Mexico, though the Delta iteration is typically made with corn meal of a coarser grind than the *masa* of the Mexican table. Some historians have guessed that Mexican field workers brought the tamales with them when they came into the region, but it is more likely that African American people borrowed the food from neighboring Native American peoples, who would have been making something like that tamale generations before the European arrival, something like I once ate in the Monacan village below Natural Bridge, Virginia, a bit of venison surrounded by coarse corn dough and then cooked in bear grease—a little heavy, but memorable.

The tamale left the Mississippi Delta around the turn of the twentieth century, sold by street vendors in Chicago, Kansas City, Los Angeles, and other venues with sizeable African American populations outside the Delta region. The famed bluesman Robert Johnson even wrote about tamales in his suggestive song "They're Red Hot," recorded in 1936 at the Gunter Hotel in San Antonio ("Hot tamales and they're red hot / yes she got 'em for sale"). The folklorist Margaret Hamilton recorded a tamer version of the song from about the same time, one that runs "Hot tamales, red hot / Two for five four for ten, / Rooster can eat 'em as well as the hen." She recalled that the tamale was, for her, long a mysterious thing, since her parents were vegetarians, so that when she finally had a taste of one, it was as if tasting forbidden fruit.

In the well-watered eastern reaches of the Southwest, rural people often made use of catfish, which sensitive diners may sometimes complain tastes like dirt but is really quite delicious. In African American communities, the catfish found favor in the weekly fish fry, a social event that often had

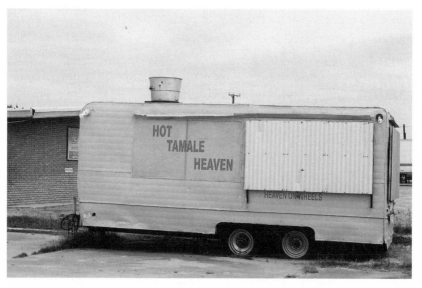

A tamale truck in Greenville, Mississippi, at the confluence of African American, Mexican, and Native American food traditions.

religious undertones, even if it also often involved a swig of whiskey or a bottle of beer as well. One of my favorite food memories is of a Fourth of July fry in Winnie, Texas, in the bayou country east of Houston. That country was still reeling from the hurricanes of 2005, but the feast was a groaning board that featured, along with innumerable kinds of macaroni salads and fruit and vegetable dishes, mounds of fried catfish, hush puppies, and alligator, all cooked in the same cornmeal and of the same shape and color. You'd never know what you were getting from one morsel to the next, but it was all very tasty and most certainly a meal for which to give thanks.

Farther West, Southern food styles found willing audiences. Toni Tipton-Martin, an Angelena who now lives in Austin and whose explorations of those styles as a cook and historian yielded the fine book *The Jemima Code: Two Centuries of African American Cookbooks*, recalls that the South was firmly rooted in the Southland. "Sweet tea and fresh-squeezed lemonade washed down Aunt Jewel's crisp fried chicken," she writes, "smoked pork bones seasoned Nannie's Sunday greens, and Mother always baked her corn bread in a big cast-iron skillet. But I didn't care for pork ribs and became easily nauseated by the potent smell of chitlins, which blasted through the air every time our neighbors from Tennessee opened their front door." She allows, however, that there were regional differences all the same: "Perhaps the most obvious evidence of my Western upbringing was my unapologetic admission that I sprinkled sugar on my grits."

It is to no one's credit that Arizona was as strong as any Deep South state in resisting civil rights. That helps explain the state's retrograde politics today, I think. Still, one of the finest soul restaurants I know sprang up in the late 1980s in Tucson, when a man named Roosevelt Foley retired from a long career as a chef in resorts and fine-dining establishments throughout the city. He played cards for a few hours, then decided that retirement wasn't for him and opened a little two-table place that he called the Soul Queen, serving up catfish, fried chicken, hush puppies, greens, and every other food to make a Southerner homesick. It wasn't long before he needed a bigger space, and soon Foley's, as it was nicknamed, was doing a thriving trade. Failing health forced him to close after a few years, but in that time, Foley introduced countless southern Arizona diners to the food he had grown up with in southeastern Texas. I like to think that every town in the region has had someone like Roosevelt Foley, an Amtrak cook or line chef or hash slinger who has cooked someone else's menu for too long and then blossomed anew when cooking on his or her own flame.

Flame: That's the operative word, for perhaps the greatest single contribution of African American cooks to Southwestern cuisine over the centuries has been in their remaking of a Native American technique, using Old World meats, mostly, in the place of the iguanas, armadillos, and venison of old.

The Taino word that gives us "barbecue" referred to a frame constructed of green twigs and sticks on which meat was laid to smoke and dry. Whether the Taino, whom Columbus encountered in 1492, or some other indigenous people came up with this method of preparing meat for storage is unknown, but it is probably very ancient—and it was certainly known to peoples far inland, used nearly everywhere early Europeans traveled in the Americas. Borrowed from Native America, the barbecue technique found some popularity in the British Caribbean colonies, less in New England, but it came to be right at home in Virginia. Food historian Robert Moss suggests that one

East Texas Barbecue Sauce

½ cup cider vinegar
1 cup water or chicken or beef broth
1 cup ketchup or ½ cup tomato paste
⅓ cup sugar
2 tablespoons chili powder
1 tablespoon hot paprika
1 teaspoon salt
1 teaspoon black or white pepper
1 tablespoon hot sauce

Combine ingredients in a bowl, using a whisk. Heat over stove or in microwave until just boiling so that sugar can melt. Allow to cool so that the flavors can blend. This sauce, a great accompaniment to barbecue beef or pork, can be made milder or spicier to taste, though smoked meat aficionados will like the fire. Add yet more heat, and you venture into South Texas style, but the vinegar connects this sauce to African American cooking traditions of the lowland South. East Texas barbecue sauce is typically thin but not watery, but the cook should feel free to adjust the liquids to taste as well.

factor for that near-instant adaptation was the colony's overabundance of pigs, both domesticated and feral and all shades in between. Pigs are easier to raise than other kinds of livestock, mostly because a pig can be let loose to forage on its own and usually can be counted on to return home without too much trouble. This is one reason that pigs are so closely associated with the poor rural South, and, in their time, particularly with slave households, where people had to work in other employment before having the time to turn to their own agricultural pursuits.

Pork lent itself to barbecuing with supreme ease, and colonial writers were soon celebrating roasts involving "hogs roasted whole . . . under a large tree," as one young man put it in 1774. Well-to-do Virginians were particularly fond of these celebratory roasts, which fell under the purview of male slaves, usually the senior cooks in a household. Wrote Louis Hughes, born into slavery in Virginia in 1832, "Barbecue originally meant to dress and roast a hog whole, but has come to mean the cooking of a food animal in this manner for the feeding of a great company." The meaning of "barbecue," then, began to shift in the nineteenth century to mean any animal roasted for a feast, and as African American cooks moved westward with American expansion, they took the word and the technique with them.

Across the South and then the Southwest, African Americans were the chief magicians behind the art of barbecuing. A soul chef named Hubert Maybell reveals some of that art with his union of food with both economics and its, well, soulfulness: "Traditionally Southern Negroes took the cheaper cuts of the hog—ham hocks, shanks and pigs feet, and things that white people throw away like greens and chitlings and made a cuisine of them by cleaning and cooking them with skill and care. They did not call it soul then, but there was a kind of ritual significance to the food. . . . You have to remember that the cuisine was developed by people who lived in the kingdom of necessity. Soul food is usually gauged by the question, 'Is it economical?'"

Economical and delicious, though sometimes disparaged as the food of the underclass, barbecue came over time to have four major branches, each with numerous tributaries that turned on both the wood used for smoking and the condiments used in the sauce accompanying the meat. Carolina barbecue, close to the Virginia colonial original, favors hickory or oak and a sauce made of vinegar and salt, perhaps with a little tomato or, if in South Carolina, mustard. Memphis barbecue introduces the dry rub—that is, the meat is rubbed with salt, pepper, and spices before smoking and is usually not eaten with a sauce—while Kansas City barbecue trades heavily on "wet," sauce-laden meat. For its part, Texas barbecue, the Southwestern contribution to the mix, uses the dense, flavorful smoke of the mesquite tree. That is to say, West Texas or "cowboy" barbecue uses mesquite fire, for elsewhere in Texas there are barbecue dialects, so to speak, such as the market style employed by German and Czech cooks in the Hill Country and, in the more Southern-flavored stretches of the bayou country and southern coastal plain, the "East Texas" style, which is essentially that of Memphis—though don't tell a Texas barbecue chef that.

From those four chief branches, whose borders are porous and variations many, barbecue has spread throughout the nation. In the Southwest, the Texas and Kansas City branches are best represented, but all can be found, all sharing what food historian Anne Yentsch portrays as an origin story of movement: "The grilled chicken, spareribs, spicy pork, and whole range of

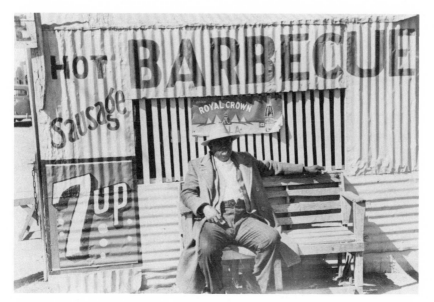

A roadside barbecue stand in Corpus Christi, Texas, 1939. Courtesy of the Library of Congress.

smoky barbecued meat cooked so well in these places—which still exist—are a continuum of the cooking that males did, beginning with those on plantations," she writes. "Steamboat cooks brought these foods up the rivers, and railroad cooks and chefs took them across the prairies."

And across the deserts and mountains, too, so that no corner of the Southwest is without its barbecue stand and the chefs who know what to do with wood, fire, smoke, and meat. Over centuries African Americans who mastered that art changed the Southern palate, and with it American—and Southwestern—cuisine. As a thoughtful writer for the British newsweekly *The Economist* puts it, "Barbecue, like jazz, develops from conversation, from talking and listening, from eating and thinking. As Duke Ellington said of music, there are really only two kinds of barbecue: good and bad." Thankfully, bad barbecue is a relative rarity, and that is thanks to the work of good cooks.

What makes soul food soul food more than anything else is its heat and other spices to enliven foods that otherwise can be a little bland or, in hard times, disguise food that might be a little off. That fire comes from New World capsicum in such forms as Scotch bonnet, malagueta, and pili-pili peppers. Add these to an otherwise uninteresting mess of limp cooked greens that whites often scorned as fodder, put in some scrap meat, and cook these with skill and care, and you have a masterpiece.

African Americans found some measure of freedom in the Southwest, and particularly California, at least as compared to the southern places they had left behind. Asked if he intended to take his earnings and leave Los Angeles to retire back home in Arkansas, the character by that name in Chester Himes's 1945 novel *If He Hollers Let Him Go* says sarcastically, "Yeah, I'm going back—when the horses, they pick the cotton, and the mules, they cut the corn; when the white chickens lay black eggs and the white folks is Jim Crowed while the black folks is—" He doesn't complete his thought, for a white foreman walks in, making even the wartime shipyards of Los Angeles a place where some thoughts are better left unexpressed.

Those shipyards, along with the railyards and aircraft factories and munitions plants of the wartime years, did much to change the face of the Southwest and with it the region's history—and indeed, its entire feel. World War II was a time of horror abroad and certainly no magical elixir at home, but it did have the effect of introducing people from all over the country and from many ethnicities in the decidedly undemocratic though oddly democratizing context of the military and the associated civilian military effort. Look at the jukebox—that resonant African term—for the year 1948, for instance, and you might think that it belonged to big bands and white pop acts alone. That year saw the debut of Redd Stewart and Pee Wee King's lovely crooner "Tennessee Waltz," with which Eddie Cochran would score a pop hit and Patsy Cline a country-chart smash a little more than a decade later. Among the nation's favorite tunes that year were Frank Loesser's "On a Slow Boat to China" and "Baby, It's Cold Outside," Kim Gannon's "I'll Be Home for Christmas," Jay Livingston and Ray Evans's "Buttons and Bows," George Morgan's "Candy Kisses," and assorted hits by the likes of The Andrews Sisters and Frank Sinatra. But in 1948 a new kind of music was also finding its way onto the airwaves and in roadside truck stops and juke joints. A blend of white and black musical forms from the Mississippi Delta, a kind of rough country music with the grinding of machinery and automobiles implicit in its grinding beat, rhythm and blues spread across the nation from its birthplace, Detroit. When white pop music entered the idiom in the immediate postwar era, rhythm and blues became rock and roll.

The same happened to food, which has always had a persistent habit of crossing color lines. And the same happened to the very idea of the Southwest, which had been a sleepy region with a stagnant economy and a culture governed by the East. After the war, its economy had diversified. So had its ethnic makeup, and all the possibilities that come from a diverse culture were suddenly the Southwest's to do with what it will. Air conditioning sealed the deal: It was suddenly possible to live in enclosed spaces and not parboil or suffocate.

African American food does not come from a single source or tradition, nor is it stagnant. It found fire in the Southwest, and it has continued to evolve here, drawing on traditions that cross the continents. Beginning in the 1980s, for example, the Southwest saw fresh waves of immigrants from Africa, including the Horn region, Darfur and South Sudan, and Ghana and Senegal. So many immigrants arrived to Los Angeles that an area of the city just north of the Art District is called Little Ethiopia. Fittingly, the newcomer communities have added many restaurants to the mix, including, of course, Ethiopian restaurants, of which there is at least one in every major Southwestern city now.

American diners have yet to know much of the African culinary tradition, but these restaurants, with varied and fascinating menus, are a start. For the moment, they offer African cuisine—but an African cuisine that is also on the way to becoming African American, and one day American writ large.

8. **The Old World and the New**

If there is a definitively Southwestern city, encompassing historical patterns and future demographic trends, it is Nogales, bridging Arizona and Sonora. Its Spanish name means "walnut trees," but it sits in an oak forest at about four thousand feet above sea level in a rugged landscape of volcanic peaks, weathered hills, and deep canyons. Come up from the south, cross Nogales at the international port of entry, as hundreds of food-bearing tractor-trailers do each day, and travel north, and you will leave the broad coastal plain of Sonora for the Gila River drainage, which drops in elevation until it hits near sea level at the junction of the Gila and the Colorado River. Cross that line today, and you run a gauntlet of metal walls and border guards, doing what both Mexico and the United States thought it unnecessary to do until recently—namely, to block the free flow of traffic between two peaceful neighbors. When Nogales was founded in the nineteenth century near the site of a series of Spanish colonial mines, a Mexican customs collector sat at one end of the canyon, an American collector at the other end, each gathering a few dollars in tariffs each day. Both collectors then repaired to the town's general store for a drink.

First came missionaries. Then came the miners—Spanish, although from the Basque-speaking regions in the northwest of

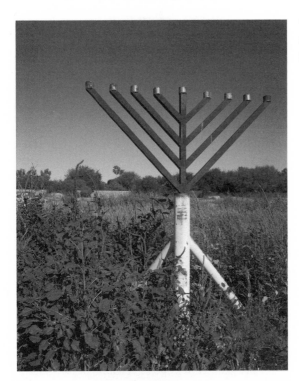

Wild amaranth grows in abundance around a menorah in Tucson.

Spain, which explains why the name Arizona should derive, perhaps improbably, from a Basque phrase meaning "place of the oaks," describing the hilly country above Nogales where the Real de Arizonac mine was situated. Then came the soldiers to protect the missionaries and miners, and then the freighters and teamsters who supplied them. Then came the merchants, and thus Nogales, a supply depot shared by two countries centered on "I. Isaacson, General Merchandise," a store owned by Isaac Isaacson, who arrived there with his brother Jacob from Russia in about 1880.

In the 1970s an archivist working with documents housed in Seville, Spain, offered a newsmaking hypothesis: Because unpublished entries in his ship's journal mention the high holidays, and because Hebrew passages sometimes occur there, it is likely that Christopher Columbus was Jewish. Add to that the fact that in the year 1492 all Jews were expelled from Spain by royal edict, and the suggestion is tempting. There is just as much evidence to suggest not, but at the very least, it is possible that several members of his crew were conversos, or Jews who had converted, willingly or not, to Christianity.

Columbus may have been among their number himself. One of his crewmembers, Luis de Torres, certainly was, and there is reason to believe that he named the bird that Columbus took back from his first voyage, calling it "*tuki*," the Hebrew word for peacock, which became our "turkey." Certainly many conversos were among those who followed Columbus into the Americas, many of whom kept the old customs even as, generation by generation, they lost memory of why they did so—why they kept Sabbath on Saturday instead of Sunday, why they lighted candles at Hanukkah, why, while their neighbors feasted on adobado, they shied away from pork. One descendant of a Sephardic family who settled at another Nogales, this the name of a ranch not far south of the Texas line in Nuevo León, recalls that this secret practice extended into the modern era:

> I was raised traditionally Jewish and was told as a child that we were
> not Catholics, and that the laws of Moses are our book, and the Old
> Testament. . . . As a child I was given by my grandmother a Hebrew
> name, Yisrael. My mother was also told to remember her Hebrew name
> and was raised learning Ladino with her grandmother . . . who also spoke
> Hebrew. . . . I inherited a gold wedding band that has been passed on
> the family with the inscription "Adonay," meaning god of the universe in
> Hebrew, a name of God.

The Jewish pioneers who followed the conversos had no need to keep their identities or their religion secret, though, and notwithstanding occasional moments of anti-Semitism—for which see Owen Wister's novel *The Virginian*—they were usually welcome or at least tolerated wherever they went. One German Jew, Isaac Lankershim, began growing wheat in the Van Nuys area in 1874. Soon he was growing wheat throughout the San Fernando Valley, with more than sixty thousand acres in cultivation, and, not coincidentally, he also owned the first flour mill in Southern California. His family's wheat farms dominated the area until 1915, when Owens Valley water began to arrive in the Los Angeles area, at which time more diversified farms sprang up in the area, growing sugar beets, melons, apricots, lettuce, avocados, and many different crops, as well as huge chicken farms. Lankershim's son sold out in 1919, ending the era of wheat production in southern California. That history is largely forgotten today, though the pioneer's name is enshrined in the major thoroughfare called Lankershim Boulevard.

A year after Lankershim's arrival, a Jewish immigrant named Isaac Goldberg, who had been successfully freighting goods to cavalry posts and mines across southern Arizona, suffered the loss of three tons of flour when a bridge collapsed. Since he was delivering a load under a federal contract, Goldberg applied for compensation. When the claim was finally settled, twenty-eight years later, he had had a storied though not entirely successful career as a merchant and miner, but, finally tired of the hard work, had moved west to California, where he died in 1902.

Escaping persecution and hunger across the ocean, Jews made substantial contributions to agriculture and food throughout the Southwest. In the southern Rio Grande Valley of New Mexico, Phoebus Freudenthal, a poultry farmer who had studied at Cornell University, introduced the pecan trees that still thrive alongside the chile fields of Hatch and Elephant Butte. Freudenthal came in the footsteps of the Spiegelberg brothers, who had developed a well-coordinated business buying vegetables and meat from farmers and ranchers throughout New Mexico and using them to supply military outposts and Indian reservations with rations.

Jews were also prominent in cattle ranching in Texas: Braise a brisket, and you have a traditional holiday dish, but smoke it, and you have the basis of Texas barbecue. An English traveler in the 1860s marveled that Americans "usually have meat three times a day, and not a small quantity at each meal either." A prominent rancher, land developer, and newspaper publisher named Jacob de Cordova, descended from a prominent Sephardic family, may have been working against his own interests when, in 1858, he advised newcomers to Texas not to be too quick to partake of all the bounty: "Beware of the excessive use of meat in summer; fat and salted meat and strong coffee clog the system. Our advice to the Northern emigrant would be, always have vegetables and fruit in plenty. . . . A decrease in meat eating, especially in hot weather, and a more liberal use of nutritious vegetables and fruit, would end a large portion of sickness among the newly arrived emigrants."

Fighting words for a Texan, that suggestion to set the T-bone aside in favor of the tangerine and turnip. At one point in the 1890s, the Halff ranch of Midland occupied two hundred thousand acres and ranked third in the

United States in livestock production, while the Levytansky ranch on the Nueces River, where Cabeza de Vaca had found provision, produced not only fine cattle but also the best olives in Texas. It was thanks to an immigrant named Isaac Dahlman that Texas became not just a place to raise cattle but also a place to process and ship them; he established commercial connections in Liverpool and elsewhere in Europe and, by way of Galveston, shipped steaks from Fort Worth across the waters. Alas, in the 1890s both the supply chain and the shipboard refrigerators were erratic, and it would be a few decades still before Fort Worth would become one of the country's preeminent cattle centers.

Still, in this land of plenty, there was plenty such work to be done. Ten thousand Jews entered the United States by way of the port of Galveston in the first decade of the twentieth century, and many remained in the Lone Star State, providing a ready market and adding to the great ethnic mix. In January 1912 Ohio-based Procter & Gamble introduced a product that, it said, was a newly discovered "ideal food," a vegetable-oil spread called Krispo. When another company objected that it made and sold crackers of that name, Procter & Gamble changed its wonder food's name to Crisco. The small company had to fight to make its new product known, for it was known as a manufacturer of industrial-strength soaps, not of food. But thanks to an ingenious campaign, Crisco became a household name in a matter of years. Among other promotional tactics, the company sent saleswomen out into communities to host "Crisco parties," featuring dishes made with the shortening. Procter & Gamble also published cookbooks of Crisco recipes—one edition featured more than six hundred items made with it—and gave away thousands of cans to grocers, who then stocked the product, which, in any event, kept better than butter and lard. Finally, the company hit on a concept we now call "niche marketing," promoting Crisco to religious groups that shunned animal fats. In all these regards, Crisco was an ideal product for kosher-keeping Jews, to whom Procter & Gamble marketed the product as something for which the "Hebrew Race" had been waiting 4,000 years."

By the 1880s, nine out of ten Jews in the United States were members of Reform congregations, with relaxed dietary laws that allowed much leeway in the personal decision of whether to keep kashrut. This proved timely, particularly in the West, where kosher meat was not easily available. One enterprising rabbi, Hyman Sharfman, traveled from Maine all the way to Corpus Christi, Texas, sometimes on horseback, teaching ranchers and settlers how to slaughter cattle and sheep in ritual accordance with Jewish law. When it developed that processors were afraid that labeling a product kosher would chase away non-Jewish customers, Sharfman invented a subtle symbol, the forerunner of the Orthodox Union hechsher, to indicate that the food was safe for observant Orthodox Jews to eat.

Throughout the Southwest most Jewish food as such was eaten at home— a familiar story before the rise of ethnic restaurants in the postwar era. Like other pioneer families Jewish Southwesterners kept chickens in their yards, but few, according to lore, as delicious as those of Charles Strauss, an early mayor of Tucson whose table was always open to hungry passersby. That generosity was widespread; Gert Silverman, raised in Nogales, recalled that the groaning board at her family's Passover Seder often fed more than fifty people, some traveling from Tucson, also a center of Southwestern Jewish life and the site of the first synagogue in Arizona.

Immigrants retained emotional bonds to some foods that had fed them in poverty, such as krupnick, a soup made of a cereal such as barley or oatmeal with potatoes and fat. Other traditional recipes for such beloved foods as latkes and roast lamb were also passed from one generation to the next, often with local and Americanized variations. Still, Crisco could not take the place of shmaltz, and here and there Jewish restaurants and delicatessens opened. One center for these was the Fairfax District of Los Angeles, northwest of the old downtown on the way to Santa Monica, where a Jewish community had existed well before the arrival of the Jews from New York, Detroit, Budapest, and other distant locales who invented the film industry. The delicatessen was a German Jewish institution, but one shaped by Eastern European preferences and the charcuterie beloved of Jews of the Alsace. A good deli provided excellent food, of course, but it also had an element of social cohesion in that it was a place where people could meet and pass time over coffee and chicken soup. It also allowed women to work, back in the day, and still have dinner waiting at the end of the day, leading one wag to remark that "the secret of a good marriage . . . was to live near a delicatessen."

The delicatessen was the place to buy many things, not least of them the bagel. The best bagels, it has to be said, come from the Habsburg heartland, where they were invented—or so legend holds—to honor the deliverance of Vienna from Ottoman siege in 1683. A Jewish Viennese baker, it seems, wanted to honor the Polish warrior king Jan Sobieski for being first on the scene, and so he concocted a roll that looked like a stirrup—in German, a *Steigbügel* or *Bügel*, shaped by the rules of Yiddish into the form *beygel*. The roll was made of white flour, then something of a luxury, and it kept well, a good thing for a knight on the march to keep in his saddlebag. It's a curiosity that *beygel* sounds very much like the Hebrew word meaning "golden calf," allowing for some spirited punning, but outside of Montreal, New York, and the Fairfax District of Los Angeles, a good bagel has proven an elusive thing in much of North America, and not just the Southwest. Even so, almost every Southwestern city with a Jewish community of any size boasts at least one good deli, adding to other testimonials to the historic Jewish presence in the region.

On the matter of baked goods, by the way, it is not too much of a stretch to think that the sopapilla, a specialty of New Mexico, where so many conversos settled early on, is a very slightly modified version of the bunuelo, fried yeast dough covered in honey, a treat that Spanish Jews traditionally eat at Hanukkah.

At about the same time that Eastern European Jews began to arrive in number in the West, so did Lebanese immigrants, most of them Maronite Christians. They often worked in the same general set of trades, operating stores and farms, and in places like Nogales there was considerable intermarriage among them and among Mexicans. One manifestation of that cultural exchange is the dish called tacos al pastor, or tacos shepherd-style, the shepherds being those Lebanese immigrants and the style spit-roasted meat, usually lamb, otherwise called shawarma. In time, most taquerias gave pork pride of place over lamb, and today a taco al pastor is a treat of spit-roasted pork that has been marinated in chile and pineapple and served on a corn tortilla with chopped onion, salsa, and cilantro, a sumptuous wedding of Middle Eastern and Mesoamerican traditions.

One Lebanese family gained prominence in the ranching business in central New Mexico. Headquartered in a little town in the hills south of Santa Rosa, now all but abandoned, the brothers Hindi, William and Alexander, married into the Duran family on arriving in New Mexico. William opened

Tacos al Pastor

Rick Bayless, originally from Oklahoma, has been studying the food of Mexico and the Southwest for decades as both anthropologist and chef, offering the results of his explorations at his famed Chicago restaurant Frontera Grill. Here is his recipe for tacos al pastor, yielding about twenty tacos.

3 ½ ounce package achiote paste
3 canned chipotle chile en adobo, plus 4 tablespoons of the canning sauce
¼ cup vegetable or olive oil, plus a little more for the onion and pineapple
1 ½ pounds thin-sliced pork shoulder
1 medium red onion, sliced ¼-inch thick
Salt
¼ medium pineapple, sliced into ¼-inch-thick rounds
20 warm corn tortillas
1 ½ cups raw tomatillo salsa

In a blender, combine the achiote paste, chiles, canning sauce, oil and ¾ cup water. Blend until smooth. Use ⅓ of the marinade to smear over both sides of each piece of meat (refrigerate the rest of the marinade to use on other meat or fish). Cover and refrigerate for at least an hour. Light a charcoal fire and let the coals burn until covered with gray ash but still very hot; bank the coals to one side and set the grill grate in place. Or, heat one side of a gas grill to high. Brush both sides of the onion slices with oil and sprinkle with salt. Lay in a single layer on the hot side of the grill. When richly browned, usually just about a minute, flip and brown the other side; move to the cool side of the grill to finish softening to grilled-onion sweetness. Oil and grill the pineapple in the same way. Finally, in batches, grill the meat: it'll take about a minute per side as well. As the meat is done, transfer it to a cutting board and chop it up (between ¼- and ½-inch pieces). Scoop into a skillet and set over the grill to keep the meat warm. Chop the onion and pineapple into small pieces as well, add them to the skillet, and toss everything together. Taste and season with salt, usually about ½ teaspoon. Serve with the tortillas and salsa for your guests to make soft tacos.

The last camp, as it's called, of Greek Muslim immigrant Hadj Ali in Quartzsite, Arizona.

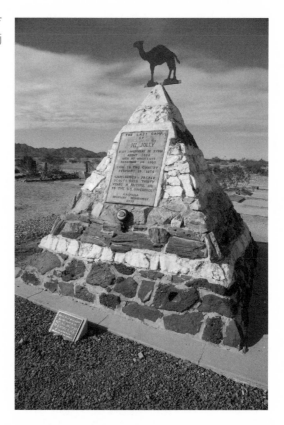

a store, the previous storeowner, another Lebanese immigrant, having been murdered, while Alexander went into the business of raising longhorn cattle, sheep, and horses. Whole lines of Arabian stock today trace their origins to the Hindi ranch.

In 1857 John B. Floyd, then the US secretary of war, imported two dozen camels from Egypt and shipped them to California, where they were put under the charge of a naval officer named Edward Beale, who had twin duties as an Indian agent and federal surveyor. Following a campaign of breeding, the camels numbered about seventy by 1859. Working with mostly Lebanese drovers, Beale used them to carry mail, supplies, and tools, more or less experimentally. Some of the camels made their way inland on expeditions, but they never fulfilled Beale's hope either of establishing a camel corps parallel to the horse cavalry or forming the basis of a camel livestock industry. After the military abandoned the experiment, the camels were turned loose in the Harquahala and Eagletail Mountains of western Arizona, from which they wandered into neighboring ranges and eventually all the way down into Mexico. It is reported that Native people were feasting on wild camels captured out in the sands up until the 1940s, making an accidental detour into the commissary of the long-distant Pleistocene. The last known wild camel died in 1956 at an oasis in Baja California.

One of those early drivers, hired at the very beginning of the experiment, was a man named Hadj Ali. He was of somewhat mysterious origin, perhaps Lebanese, perhaps Syrian, perhaps Jordanian. He also answered to the Greek name of Philip Tedro, and since seven of the other drivers brought over with him were Greek, there is reason to think that he was a Greek instead, and a Greek convert to Islam at that. Known as Hi Jolly to his neighbors along the Colorado River, Hadj Ali worked as a drover and guide, marrying into the Mexican Serna family and ending his days in the low desert town of Quartzsite, where he made a few dollars in his later years by selling camel jerky to hungry travelers in the desert. After his death in 1902—he was out hunting wild camels at the time—a pyramidal monument went up over his supposed burial site, though, as with Billy the Kid, it's said that Hi Jolly really lies elsewhere.

One of Hadj Ali's fellow drovers, known as Greek George, was implicated in a crime in southern California and hanged for his troubles. The murderer of William Hindi's predecessor in Duran was hanged, too—the last man to be hanged in New Mexico, in fact. Greeks and Lebanese figure prominently in the region's history, and it's no accident that their cuisines are abundantly represented throughout the Southwest.

Not far from Quartzsite lies the little Colorado River town of Ehrenberg, Arizona, named for a curious character in Arizona history. Born in 1816, Hermann Ehrenberg was a German mining engineer who had seen much adventure in his day, having fought in the Texas War of Independence and written of it for the European press after he returned home to Germany. He came to the United States again in the early 1840s and traveled by way of the Oregon Trail to the Pacific, where he proceeded on to Hawaii and Polynesia before landing in the Southwest, where he mapped the newly acquired territory of the Gadsden Purchase and undertook several mining ventures. He, too, was murdered in 1866 at the stagecoach station at Mecca, California, while carrying gold to San Diego. A Jewish immigrant merchant on the Colorado River, a friend of Ehrenberg's named Michael Goldwater, grandfather of Barry, named the town site in his honor.

Germans had begun to arrive in Sonora and southern California—largely an outpost of Sonora—in number in the 1830s, where they worked as bakers and brewers and established the Mexican brewing industry. In 1857 German farmers established a utopian colony at a place along the Santa Ana River that they called Anaheim, near the site of another utopia, Disneyland. Following political unrest in Mexico in the 1870s and 1880s, still more Germans came north into the Southwest. One of them was the son of a German immigrant named Friedrich August Ronstadt, who came to Mexico in the 1840s. Born in Banámichi, Sonora, Federico José María Ronstadt arrived in Tucson in 1882 and established a successful carriage business, branching out into hardware and machinery and becoming a central figure in the city's business and political communities. When he was not working, Frederick, as he was now known, played in a brass band in a German-style beer garden where sausage and tamales were sold side by side—and where, the story has it, a dancing bear entertained guests, a bear whose ghost can still be seen dancing among the cottonwoods. Frederick's granddaughter Linda carried the family name forward in the music business, as have other supremely talented descendants.

Germans were nowhere better represented than in Texas, however. Beginning in the 1830s and 1840s freethinking German immigrants left a place of political turmoil and oppression and moved to what was celebrated as the freest land in the world. Moving into the Hill Country and establishing towns such as New Braunfels and Fredericksburg, where German was the first language within living memory, they brought their cuisine and traditions with them. Those hallmarks influenced and were in turn influenced by neighboring traditions, so that Mexican *norteño* music is quite obviously polka with a different accent, while Texas-style chili can be thought of as a Hungarian goulash brought over by German cooks who found a pepper hotter even than paprika. In that light, the beloved Texas concoction known as the chicken fried steak is simply wiener schnitzel, or Viennese-style breaded cutlet, translated to a new continent but renamed

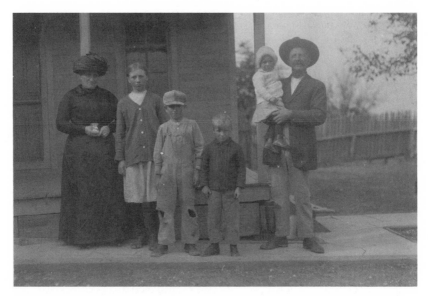

A Czech immigrant family in Texas in about 1913. Courtesy of the Library of Congress.

to disguise its German origins during a period of anti-German sentiment that accompanied and followed World War I. Even as late as 1943, however, Texas cookbooks still called it by its original name, even as towns throughout the Hill Country and the South Plains vied to be recognized as the birthplace of Texas-style chicken fried steak, an honor that probably should be split between Lamesa, Bandera, and Boerne.

Czechs figure as well in the food history of Texas, adding kolaches (a dish that *Texas Monthly* writer Courtney Bond gamely calls "Czexan") and sausages to the larder and trading with neighboring traditions as well, which explains the hybrid festival called Czhilispiel celebrated each year in Flatonia, a Czech town near Praha and Moravia, not far from Rosanky and Kovar—and Winchester, Gonzalez, La Grange, and McMahan. Danes put Solvang, California, on the map in what is now the state's southern wine belt. Travelers passing through there on the way to places bearing such names as Lompoc, Betteravia, and Los Angeles know to stop for a bowl of delicious pea soup, though they may not always know what ethnic tradition they are commemorating.

Kolache

Kolache is a beloved Czech *svacina*, or midday snack, that in Texas became a treat suitable for consumption at just about any time of day. Texan travelers to the mother country, it's said, come home pining for the Lone Star version of the baked good, which tends to be stuffed to overstuffedness with good things such as fruit, cheese, and meat. This version, adapted from the Little Czech Cafe in West, is based on locally grown apricots.

12 ounces dried apricots
3 tablespoons unsalted butter
½ teaspoon almond extract
½ cup sugar
½ cup + 1 tablespoon sugar
1 tablespoon + 1 teaspoon active dry yeast
2 cups warm water
2 cups milk
2 cups vegetable shortening
3 teaspoons salt
2 egg yolks, beaten
6 cups + ⅓ cup sifted all-purpose flour
1 stick unsalted butter, melted

Cover the apricots with boiling water, allowing them to rehydrate. Let sit until cold, preferably overnight. In a saucepan, melt butter, then warm the apricots, blending in the almond extract and sugar. Mash the cooked fruit with a whisk or potato ricer, or purée it in a food processor. Set aside to cool.

Mix 1 tablespoon sugar, 1 tablespoon yeast, and warm water. Warm the milk and stir in shortening. Remove from heat and allow to cool, then place in a large bowl and add salt, egg yolks, and ½ cup sugar and blend with a whisk. Add yeast mixture and stir. Add the flour, working it with a wooden spoon until it forms a soft, stretchy dough. Cover the bowl with a towel and let the dough rise for an hour. When the dough has risen, punch it down to remove excess air.

Flour a cutting board and, with a spoon, drop spoonfuls of dough onto it. Using your palms, roll the dough out into balls the size and shape of eggs. Lay these out on greased cookie sheets and brush with melted butter. Then, with a spoon, press out a hole in the center of each dough ball and fill with the apricot mixture. Top the dough with brown sugar or sugar mixed with butter. Let it rise again for an hour and then bake at 375 degrees for about 25 minutes.

Not so with the food of the French-speaking Acadians, or Cajuns, who are central to Louisiana's identity but just as important in the history and culture of southeastern Texas. French food is not, as a categorical statement, notably piquant, but Cajun cooking certainly is, a difference that can be attributed to the proximity of Latin America—which also explains why tamales should appear on Cajun menus alongside alligator (*el lagarto*, that is, "the lizard" in Spanish), andouille sausage, and crawdaddies. Farther west, French speakers also introduced Los Angeles to the finer sort of dining: in the mid-1850s a French immigrant named Jean La Rue opened the first true restaurant in the city, even if historians Leonard Pitt and Dale Pitt describe it as "a scruffy, mud-floor, one-room" affair. French cuisine was the standard for high-end, sit-down restaurants in the decades afterward, and even today places ranging from the low-end Original Pantry in downtown to far fancier venues on Rodeo Drive offer French or French-inspired fare—including the French dip sandwich, of course, which originated in the kitchen of Philippe, a French restaurant that opened in Los Angeles in 1908.

The first Italian restaurants in the West—and among the first in the United States, period—were founded in San Francisco, attached to boardinghouses and hotels that catered to newly arrived immigrants, almost all of them young men. Known more for quantity than quality, they nevertheless served meals that reminded the newcomers of home. Soon Italian bakeries sprang up in the city, founded by gold miners who, eschewing the corn bread and sourdough of the Americans and the tortillas of the Mexicans, built makeshift beehive ovens in the goldfields to bake crusty pane. As Italian communities began to form in the city and, later, in Los Angeles, they often did so around these pioneering food suppliers.

Italians were no strangers to the interior West. With a few outliers such as Scordato's in Tucson and Pietro's in Dallas, though, it would seem that they did their best cooking at home. It was a product of critical mass that the situation began to change in the 1980s, when enough Southwesterners had traveled to Italy and tasted real pasta and real coffee that a sustainable market opened up. It's still not easy to find a pizza beyond the unconvincing offerings of the chains in many Southwestern towns, but at least it's more possible than it was just a few years ago. As a member of northwestern European tribes that, as food historian Hasia Diner observes, did not bother to "fuse food and ethnic identity," I have been one of countless beneficiaries of the Italian presence, among other cultures from continental Europe and many other places besides that took food as more than just a vehicle for staying alive.

Nogales, known for its first few years as Isaacson, is the definitive Southwestern city indeed. Charles Mingus, the great African American jazz musician, was born there, the son of a "buffalo soldier." Chinese, Asian Indian, and Filipino merchants lived and worked there. As with cities much larger, at least one of every kind of person—Jew, Slav, Irish, Mexican, Native American, Greek, Lebanese—has lived there at one time or another, or so it seems. Cosmopolitan and culturally connected to several major cities, among them Los Angeles and Mexico City, it was a magnet for rural Southwesterners, a path to novelty and different futures.

But as for the recent past, before the border was tightened to protect us from Nicaraguan tanks and hordes of Arab terrorists, it was an easy matter to stroll across the border and stumble back after a meal at one of the restaurants owned by the city's Greek-Jewish-German-Mexican first families. Other such families settled across the line and opened restaurants, my favorite of which offers "Mexican caviar"—refried beans, that is—and gyro meat spiced with chiles.

It is fitting that Nogales native Alberto Ríos, the eminent poet and novelist, should have entitled his 1999 memoir *Capirotada*, evoking a kind of bread pudding beloved by people on both sides of the border. But let him tell it:

> *Capirotada*: This is indeed simply a bread pudding, but it would be unfair to stop there in the description. "Bread pudding" says so little about it, as so many words are unequal to their task. Made with a zoo of foods, each thing in it is good, but taken together *capirotada* is Mexican cooking's version of fruitcake, but raised several notches to the level of a one-ring circus, with everybody and everything gathered at the grand finale. It assembles into the single ring at the center, and in view of the full spotlight, all the star performers, the high-wire walkers, the

elephants and clowns, beasts from the far ends of the cooking cosmos: prunes and peanuts, white bread, raisins, milk, *quesadilla* cheese, butter, cinnamon and cloves, old world sugar. All this, and those things people will not tell you.

Those things people will not tell you: Those are the things of which history and stories are made, the things we are beholden and honor-bound to find for ourselves if we are to carry them into the future.

9. **Asian Americans**

Allowing for the Ice Age, migrants from eastern Siberia—the first Asians to arrive in the Southwest—came by sea. Filipinos who put ashore at Morro Bay (north of present-day Santa Barbara) in 1587 were members of a galleon crew who, while plying the Manila-to-Acapulco trade, had been pushed far off course by a storm. Eight years later a second Filipino galleon crew would be shipwrecked at Point Reyes (north of present-day San Francisco)—though, this time, the survivors were rescued and returned home. Small numbers of "Manilamen" would arrive over the years, many settling on the Gulf Coast of Texas and in western Louisiana and some even serving in the Confederate Navy during the Civil War.

The first Asians to come in number were the Chinese, who arrived at the place they called Gold Mountain—California—in 1849, following the discovery of gold at Sutter's Mill and the subsequent rush of migrant miners from every part of the world. No sooner had the Chinese arrived than a restaurant opened in San Francisco, and soon small Chinese diners popped up among the gold camps, introducing European and American miners to such things as dumplings for breakfast and curious kitchen-sink dishes making use of whatever was available, which would give rise to the Americanized one-pot meal called chop suey. In its earliest iteration that dish was not for the squeamish; one scrupulous American diner in the 1880s reported that it contained tripe, gizzards, livers, and other organ meats, as well as "various other ingredients which I was unable to make out." That notwithstanding, the diner allowed that the dish was very good, if "of a mysterious nature." And if another Anglo Californian had complained twenty years earlier that Chinese food was served "in a sort of hash form" that tended to taste the same from dish to dish, another praised the newcomers: "They serve everything promptly, cleanly, hot, and well cooked." The first Chinese restaurants in San Francisco, wrote *New York Tribune* correspondent Bayard Taylor in 1849, were "much frequented by Americans, on account of their excellent cookery, and the fact that meals are $1 each, without regard for quantity. Kong-Sung's house is near the water; Wang-Tong's in Sacramento Street; and Tong-Ling's in Jackson Street. There the grave Celestials serve up their chow-chow and curry, besides many genuine English dishes; their tea and coffee cannot be surpassed."

Soon Chinese workers were laboring alongside Americans, Mexicans, Europeans, and African Americans on the railroad crews lacing California with rail lines, and as railhead towns were established farther inland, in Arizona and New Mexico and Texas, small settlements of Chinese began to dot the West. Some of these "Chinatowns," as they were known, came to be large and heavily trafficked by non-Chinese seeking meals and supplies. In mining towns such as Prescott, Arizona, and railhead and port cities such as Tucson and Houston, Chinese migrants became merchants, farmers, grocers, and especially restaurateurs, and almost every town in the region of any size soon had a place selling Chinese dishes of various sorts. Praised for their cooking skills, they were also often hired as domestic staff, competing with Irish and Eastern European arrivals, which led to countless incidents of strife among immigrant groups.

The farther into the interior the Chinese went, the heavier their cooking became: the delicate, lightly dough-wrapped tidbits variously called eggrolls or spring rolls, for instance, became thick, deep-fried footballs inland. Only recently have their lighter cousins become widely available outside of Los Angeles and San Francisco. I have an idle theory about this, namely that the Chinese who cooked for predominantly American audiences tried to give them what they were used to: heavy, fried foods served with gloppy sauces and lots of starch. Certainly that describes most of what passed for Chinese food away from the coasts until only recently. There were exceptions, of course; one of my happier food memories is a meal at a Chinese restaurant deep inside the Navajo Nation in northeastern Arizona, where a group of medical residents at the Indian Health Service hospital had pooled their resources and hired a chef from San Francisco. When the students completed their government obligation, the Tuba City restaurant closed, but for a few brilliant years it was a haven for hungry *Bilagáana* and Diné alike.

Chinese feasts can be elaborate affairs, but perhaps none more so than the legendary one served up for Schuyler Colfax, then Speaker of the US House of Representatives, who visited San Francisco in 1865 to thank California for remaining loyal to the Union. At a restaurant in Chinatown he was served anywhere from a dozen to nearly twelve dozen separate dishes—the accounts vary wildly—that included shark's fin, pigeon's nest soup, pig ears, stewed duck, oysters, pickled vegetables, and "a fungus-like moss" that history has yet to identify.

We might admire Colfax's adventurous palate today, but such feasts, promoted by a business association, were rare excursions into exotica in his time. It would not be until the postwar era that Chinese food became something that non-Chinese diners sought, although it was long a favorite of Jews in part because it was available on Christian holidays when stores and restaurants were closed for business.

In the catch-as-catch-can setting of the frontier West, some of the old ideals of Chinese food were sacrificed in any event. The classic *Book of the Yellow Emperor* calls for a regime of balance, with the fruit of five trees, the flesh of five animals, and the five classical vegetables providing nourishment, not just a balanced meal but a symphony of complementary tastes and values. Meat, typically used as a garnish in a diet favoring fresh vegetables, became a disproportionately dominant part of the meal, reflecting the tastes of the larger society. Until the advent of modern refrigeration and transport networks, green vegetables and fruits were seasonally unavailable, while such delicacies as seaweed were not to be found inland. Still, Chinese cooks made do. The old joke that Han tell of Cantonese and Cantonese tell of Han, "They'll eat anything that flies except an airplane and anything with four legs except a table," applied to their situation.

Even if canned mushrooms and sadly boiled chicken were often the order of the day, Chinese restaurants were prized for their inexpensive offerings and wide selection of menu choices—including, in most South-western cities, American and Mexican dishes. The Chinese immigrants themselves were not so well liked. Anti-Chinese riots and violence were commonplace throughout the West, and beginning in the 1870s numerous exclusion acts were passed that barred Chinese from working and living in many municipalities and from owning property. Newspapers calumniated against Chinese restaurants and laundries. One California editor thundered, "Do you not know that (in these exciting times when the Chinese are losing employment, and naturally mad at the white race) you are taking desperate chances of having disease introduced among us that will render desolate our firesides?" Another California newspaper described Chinese as "half-human, half-devil, rat-eating, rag-wearing, law-ignoring, Christian-civilization-hating, opium-smoking, labor-degrading, entrail-sucking Celestials." Chinese produce was also shunned, since it was grown with night soil and "every imaginable kind of filth." Even so, the quality of the goods from Chinese gardens, including more exotic items such as lichee, kumquat, bitter melons, and the like, kept plenty of "Celestial" farmers in business.

Pineapple Salsa

Mexicali-style Chinese-Mexican fusion food is beginning to make its way north of the border, with outliers throughout the Central Valley and, now, Los Angeles and Las Vegas. Look for more "Chinexican" outposts in the coming years. Meanwhile, this recipe for pineapple salsa blends ingredients from around the world as an accompaniment to grilled fish, seafood, or fowl.

1 tablespoon grapeseed oil
30 ounces diced pineapple
1 small red onion, minced
1 small habanero pepper, minced
6 ounces fresh lemon juice
2 teaspoons sea salt

In a skillet, preheat oil. Add pineapple and cook for five minutes. Remove from pan. Mix the other ingredients, then add the cooked pineapple.

Curiously, given its recent history of ethnic lawmaking, Arizona was a comparative haven for Chinese immigrants throughout the late nineteenth century. Wyatt Earp and his band of rustlers turned lawmen who rustled on the side frequented the Can Can Restaurant, founded in Tombstone by a Hong Kong immigrant named Quong Gee Kee, who said of one of the unfortunate Clantons gunned down at the OK Corral, "Nice boy, always paid his bills." Until the mines closed in the late 1880s, Kee operated three restaurants in Tombstone and nearby towns, and on his death in 1936 he was honored as one of the few non-Anglos to be buried in the town's famed Boot Hill Cemetery. By the same token, until the 1960s, most groceries in Tucson were owned by Chinese families. More than ninety were in operation in the 1940s, though only a handful remain.

Elsewhere in the Southwest, the Chinese presence was similarly marked. The Chinese population of El Paso, Texas, numbered only about seven hundred in 1890, but Chinese merchants and restaurateurs were doing a thriving trade. Still, a final exclusion act in 1882 touched off a movement not just to ban Chinese immigration but also to deport Chinese who were already in the United States, resulting in a test of the Fourteenth Amendment guarantee of birthright citizenship that was argued all the way up to the Supreme Court thanks to the persistence of an American-born Chinese chef named Wong Kim Ark. The Court ruled in his favor in 1898, but it did not end the racial enmity he encountered, and Ark moved to his family's ancestral China soon after, never to return to the United States. Chinese were banned from becoming naturalized citizens until as late as 1943, while a vigilante group that rode the Southwestern border to keep Chinese from crossing the desert evolved into what became the Border Patrol. It was not until after World War II that Chinese and other Asians were permitted to enter the country in number, and when that happened, thousands of newcomers introduced a new wave of restaurants and farms to the region; Texas in particular saw an explosion of Chinese immigrants and, in turn, restaurants in the 1970s, particularly in San Antonio and Houston but also, to a smaller extent, in the old foothold of El Paso.

Mexico was friendlier than the United States during those years of exclusion, and many Chinese chose to settle in northern Baja California rather than be subjected to the discriminatory laws north of the border. It is for that reason that Mexicali, a city of nearly a million residents just south of the international line, is today a center of New World Chinese cooking, with more than two hundred Chinese restaurants. Like offshoots in nearby El Centro, California, these restaurants offer a wonderful fusion of Chinese and Mexican cooking, with dishes such as arrachera (minced beef) with asparagus in black bean sauce and fried chiles in lemon sauce.

Another possible instance of fusion is not well documented, but it makes good sense. The concoction called the chimichanga, which we met earlier, has been claimed by restaurants in Arizona and New Mexico, but it almost certainly originated in Sonora or Sinaloa. One Mexican scholar believes that the dish was an approximation of a Chinese egg roll, for both Mexican states were heavily populated by Chinese immigrants, almost all of them men, in the early years of the twentieth century. Often these Chinese men married Mexican women, whose work in the kitchen would in turn produce the wedding of cuisines that produced the *chivichanga*—a word that could be a Mexican Spanish approximation for a Chinese name for the treat.

Japanese began to arrive in California not long after the close of the Civil War, with the first arriving to take part in a utopian religious colony in Santa Rosa—a California thing, one might say, recalling the Germans of Anaheim. Though they faced exclusion and discrimination as well, including a so-called gentleman's agreement of 1907 that kept Japanese laborers from leaving their homeland for the United States, these immigrants proved immensely skilled at the irrigated agriculture that characterized the interior Southwest, by which widespread grain cultivation gave way to fruit and vegetable crops.

One native son, a first-generation Japanese American named Toshio Mori, described the Japanese community he grew up in both at home and in internal exile at an internment camp in Utah in his 1949 book *Yokohama, California*. In one odd passage, he describes the prelude to an odd, bibulous encounter that would devolve into an argument about eggs, with the drinker in question declaring that, in the end, the egg is "the most important and the most disturbing thing in the world."

I was at Mr. Hasegawa's when Sessue Matoi staggered in the house with several drinks under his belt. About the only logical reason I could think of for his visit that night was that Sessue Matoi must have known that Mr. Hasegawa carried many bottles of Japanese-imported sake. There was no other business why he should pay a visit to Mr. Hasegawa's. I knew Mr. Hasegawa did not tolerate drinking bouts. He disliked riotous scenes and people.

The Japanese who arrived in the Southwest, most in California, valued order and hard work, and although they encountered plenty of racist opposition, they were generally valued for their contributions to the local economy. By the turn of the twentieth century, the issei and nisei, first- and second-generation immigrants, were producing nearly three quarters of California's valuable strawberries, and a generation later their sansei descendants were growing almost all of California's celery and snap beans and two-thirds of the state's tomato crop. Similarly high productivity marked Japanese farms elsewhere in the Southwest, and when many of these were expropriated or legally encumbered during the terrible years of internment during World War II (for which, among other sources, see the film *Bad Day at Black Rock*), the region's agriculture suffered accordingly.

Japanese cuisine is varied and supremely sophisticated, reckoned by gourmands and chefs as one of the world's great culinary traditions. Yet Japanese food took a long time to enter the American mainstream, and when it did, it happened with a perhaps unlikely vehicle along a likely avenue. After World War II many Americans returned from the Pacific theater with Japanese brides and a taste for their food. In the small Little Tokyo section of Los Angeles and the Miyako Restaurant in downtown San Diego—favored by American sailors and marines—but almost nowhere else could one find curious dishes made of vinegared rice and raw fish. This sushi, as it was called, was a kind of Japanese fast food whose origins can be traced to the year 1824, when a Tokyo food vendor began to make these bite-sized treats by hand—*nigiri*, that is—for hurried customers, a handful of pressed rice here and a thin slab of fish there. Yohei Hanaya's innovation spawned a legion of imitators, and nigiri sushi then as now was a popular snack.

American military personnel in Japan brought a liking for sushi back from Japan with them, and it was through their influence that sushi spread into the Southwest and then into the larger nation. Ground zero was Tucson, where an immigrant from Chihuahua, Gene Sanchez, had returned from service in the Air Force with a Japanese bride named Michiko, nicknamed Michi. After he left the service, Gene opened a shop selling Japanese imported goods and

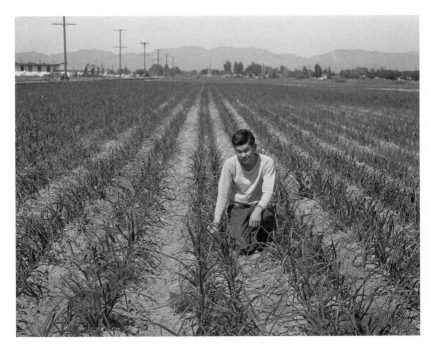

A Japanese American farmer works an onion field in Los Angeles in 1942, just before being sent to an internment camp. Courtesy of the Library of Congress.

small appliances, and in the small back room of his Tokyo Store, Michi would serve sushi on weekend nights. I celebrated my twenty-fifth birthday there in 1982 with a small crowd of journalist friends, filling the dozen or so seats. By my twenty-sixth birthday the word had spread, and Gene and Michi were serving sushi in a larger room seating thirty or so diners. Within a year they had opened three sushi restaurants, bringing in assistant chefs from Japan to help Michi. Within another year, there were at least two dozen sushi restaurants in the city—one of them opened by a Mexican couple of Japanese descent, who served up a sobering line of nigiri laced with chiles.

Elsewhere in the Southwest, the story is the same: Military personnel, usually connected to the Air Force, sustained a Japanese-owned small restaurant that gained in popularity to the point that sushi attained the status of fad. In the mid-1980s the number of Japanese restaurants throughout the United States quintupled. Many failed as the fad played out, but many remain. According to Hirotaka Matsumoto, a Japanese restaurateur and student of food trends, of the twenty-five thousand or so Japanese restaurants outside Japan, fully two-thirds serve sushi. Many of the rest are Japanese steakhouses—a genre popularized by an immigrant named Rocky Aoki, who in 1964 founded the once immensely popular Benihana chain, with an outlet in nearly every major city in the Southwest.

Sushi long ago lost its connotation of working-class, cheap snack, but it offers a nice illustration of scarcity and making do all the same. In the post-war era Japanese fish vendors promoted tuna belly, earlier used as fatty scrap for broth and for cat food, which became a status item at a premium price. Following the atomic tests in the Pacific that gave rise to the *Godzilla* film industry, tuna and other food fish became even scarcer in the region, and sushi allows for a broad distribution of small pieces of the fish to a broad audience just as efficiently and more interestingly than a can of tuna fish. Japanese cooks long ago mastered the use of reconstituted, extruded, or otherwise frankensteined fish involving the blanching of fish and processing of its protein in forms that the food industry calls "seafood analogues"—imitation crab and lobster, for instance. The United States is a leader in producing what gourmands dismiss as "fake fish," using Alaskan pollock as the most common base—but now that pollock is scarce thanks to overfishing and pollution, we may see other forms of that protein in nigiri in the near future.

Sushi has proved as successful a Southwestern export as the taco, though the critical role of the region in spreading the Japanese wonder is too little acknowledged. A similar success story also concerns a Japanese product that entered by way of California, the ramen noodle. A staple of Chinese cuisine, ramen, born lo mein, had become popular in Japan thanks to a Chinese fast food fad that had swept Japan in the 1910s. After World War II, with food and cooking oil in short supply, a Taiwanese immigrant to Japan named Ando Momofuku developed a way to dry soup mixes that leveraged abundant surplus flour supplied by the US occupation forces. "I pondered how to mass-produce ramen and give it a homemade flavor," Ando recalled, eventually hitting on the right formula. Though generations of poor students in the United States and Britain have merely endured the ubiquitous ramen noodle soup, it has proven both a culinary and a technological triumph that, Ando would insist, saved traditional Japanese food culture by diverting that flour from the production of alien bread to the production of noodles.

It's worth recalling in passing on this note that a similar noodle-based story emerged from the Italian theater of the war. When GIs arrived in 1943 to battle the forces of Fascist Italy and Nazi Germany, they brought with them abundant stocks of powdered eggs and dehydrated bacon, goods that served as a currency of goodwill—and sometimes actual currency—in a starving nation. Combined with pasta, these ingredients became pasta carbonara, the name suggesting food that one might feed a hungry coal miner in need of ample sustenance before heading into the pit, rather as a transcontinental railroad builder might open the day with a heavy English breakfast prepared by a Chinese cook.

The Filipino presence has long been strong in the Southwest, particularly in California, where fieldworkers from the islands provided much of the agricultural labor in the Central Valley until the arrival of Mexican workers in the 1930s, the so-called braceros. Filipino immigrant Carlos Bulosan arrived in California during the Depression and did odd jobs and restaurant work until becoming an itinerant farmworker, hopping the rails to the next harvest. In his 1946 book *America Is in the Heart*, he describes the feeling of jumping on a midnight special:

> I wanted suddenly to go back to Stockton and look for a job in the tomato fields, but the train was already traveling fast. . . . I could see the faint blaze of Stockton's lights in the distance, a halo arching above it and fading into a backdrop of darkness.
>
> In the early morning the train stopped a few miles from Miles, in the midst of a wide grape field. The grapes had been harvested and the bare vines were falling to the ground. The apricot trees were leafless. Three railroad detectives jumped out of a car and ran toward the boxcars. I ran to the vineyard and hid behind a smudge pot, waiting for the next train from Stockton. A few bunches of grapes still hung on the vine, so I filled my pockets and ran for the tracks when the train came.

With Filipinos, South Asians have been present in the Southwest in small numbers for decades. The partition of India and Pakistan roughly coincided with a modest relaxation of immigration restrictions for people from the region in the late 1940s, and soon pockets of settlement sprang up in California and the Texas cities of Dallas and Houston, augmented by new arrivals

California Roll

The California roll is a perfect illustration of how cultural traditions can be so smoothly blended that, not long after, it seems as if they had always been around. It dates to the very early 1960s and to a sushi restaurant in the Little Tokyo district of downtown Los Angeles, where a chef known to history only as Mr. Mashita pondered how to lure in American diners who had qualms about eating raw fish. (An alternate version of the story calls the chef Manashita.) He took a little cooked crab, combined it with cucumber and avocado, which had the pleasing oiliness of raw tuna, and then reversed the order of the traditional sushi roll, so that the vinegared rice was on the outside and the seaweed wrapper on the inside. The avocado made the name "California roll" seem wholly natural, and though Mr. Mashita's restaurant is long gone, his invention has spread throughout the United States, and even to restaurants in Japan that cater to a Western clientele.

1 ½ cups short-grain rice
Small piece of sea kelp
4 sheets toasted seaweed
2 tablespoons rice vinegar
2 tablespoons sugar
1 teaspoon salt
1 ½ teaspoon toasted sesame seeds
1 cucumber, cut lengthwise into eight pieces
1 ripe avocado, sliced lengthwise into thin pieces
8 ounces crabmeat

Cook rice with sea kelp. In a small bowl, combine vinegar, salt, and sugar and let solids dissolve. Add mixture to rice.

Using a sushi mat and plastic wrap, lay sheet of seaweed down and spread one quarter of the rice mixture. Sprinkle with sesame seeds. Lengthwise, lay down a cucumber slice, then avocado, then crabmeat, then another cucumber slice. Roll and cut with a sharp knife into bite-sized pieces.

in the 1960s, when those restrictions were largely lifted. Beginning in the 1990s, a time of economic transformation, South Asian immigrants also arrived in number in Phoenix and Albuquerque, many with connection to high-technology industries and academia.

Before the 1940s South Asians came to the Southwest in small numbers, often by way of South America, Canada, and the Caribbean, where they had worked in British colonial enterprises before finding their way into the United States. Many settled in the San Joaquin Valley of California and worked in agriculture. Barred by racial laws from marrying whites, these South Asians typically married into Mexican families, giving rise to a vanishingly small census category that has been called "Punjabi Mexicans." Small communities of these people can be found in Phoenix and in Mexicali and neighboring El Centro—the last the site of a gurdwara, or Sikh religious center. Punjabi Mexicans faced discrimination, of course, but they forged strong communities bound by marriage and custom in agricultural centers such as Casa Grande, Arizona, where Amelia Singh Netervala fondly recalls her mother's curry enchiladas as a delicious symbol of her twinned lineage. "Looking back—when you're young, you don't appreciate or realize the wealth that the two cultures brought together," she told a writer for the *Washington Post*. "But, if you'd ask me, I'd say the Punjabi-Mexican community is distinctly American."

That's just right. South Asian restaurants can now be found throughout the Southwest, especially in Southern California and the larger cities. Increasingly, though, they are turning up in small towns along the old US highways such as the storied Route 66, where South Asians—particularly members of a Gujarati subcaste named Patel—have been buying and renovating old hotels for the last couple of decades. The first Indian hotel owner in the country was an immigrant named Kanjibhai Desai, who pulled together his scant savings to purchase the Goldfield Hotel in downtown San Francisco in the early 1940s. Two decades later there were still only five dozen or so Indian-owned hotels in the country, almost all in California. That began to change in the 1970s, and today it is estimated that fully half the hotels and motels in the United States are owned by South Asian immigrants and, increasingly, their first-generation Asian American children. This phenomenon is marked by signs reading "American-Owned" in hotels throughout the Southwest, a quietly insistent and fundamentally unpleasant suggestion that the newcomers are not American, as might be gauged by the strange smells coming from their kitchens.

But thus ever it has been, a tale of strange smells that have become familiar and even assimilated—sometimes to the point of becoming passé and forgotten. For instance, the Asian fare that was common when I was a child, dominated by Chinese dishes such as chow mein, egg foo young, and chop suey, is now largely extinct. Many Chinese restaurants in the United States are now operated by Fujianese, rather than the Cantonese of previous generations, and if their menus are not terribly daring, they dependably offer dishes that have themselves become American favorites: egg rolls, lo mein, mu shu pork, General Tso's chicken. These, in time, will also become familiar and will then be forgotten, even as new dishes enter the culinary lexicon.

More adventurous venues are widely available. In my hometown of Tucson there are a couple of restaurants serving Yunnanese food, while my favorite is staffed by immigrants from Shanghai, a city that ranks among my favorite food destinations anywhere in the world. But Asian cuisine is much more than Chinese food. We have only begun to explore its manifold possibilities.

Restrictions against Asian immigration, shameful though they were, did not begin to lift until the 1970s. With the collapse of South Vietnam in 1975, a wave numbering many thousands of immigrants entered the country, most of them well-educated people associated with the South Vietnamese government in some way. The blue-collar "boat people" of the late 1970s, fleeing the communist regime, added to their number. Against considerable local opposition, many of these newcomers settled in Texas, where the Gulf Coast was a reminder, in climate and vegetation, of the country they had left behind. By the 1990s Houston ranked second only to Los Angeles in the number of immigrant Vietnamese living there, and by that time the Vietnamese had become integral to the state's fishing industry, though not without tension among the long-established Cajun fishing people of the coast. Several thousand Vietnamese settled in places such as Phoenix and Albuquerque, bringing with them their food traditions. Perhaps because of the difficulty in resettling among sometimes-hostile neighbors who did not care to be reminded of military defeat in Vietnam, these communities often seemed to exhibit a fortress mentality. When, in the mid-1980s, the writer Charles Bowden and I used to duck into a Tucson eatery called the Three

Sisters, we were regarded with considerable (and probably justifiable) suspicion by diners who favored mirrored sunglasses indoors or out and who chain-smoked between the endless parade of dishes placed before them.

Since that time, however, Vietnamese communities have come to be more at home throughout the Southwest, and most cities have one or more Vietnamese restaurants, including, recently, ones that serve pho, a kind of Vietnamese soup made of beef and rice noodles that originated in the countryside near Hanoi. Vendors in the old country sold the soup from cauldrons carried over the shoulder at the ends of a bamboo pole called a *ganh pho*, and in time, by one theory, the transporting device became the name of the thing it carried. Another theory has it that the name is an approximation of the kindred French dish pot-au-feu, with which the soup has visible kinship. Growing in popularity in communities with substantial Vietnamese populations are casual restaurants that serve banh mi, "bread." These sandwiches resemble the Cajun po' boy in using a white-flour baguette as the delivery vehicle for a variety of cold cuts and vegetables—usually pickled vegetables, in the case of banh mi, and with chili sauce as a condiment, a blend of hot and cold that is right in keeping with long-established Southwestern food tastes.

In much the same way, Thai food has become widely popular throughout the United States, and most Southwestern cities have at least one Thai restaurant and sometimes many more. These restaurants are sometimes in unlikely places. One of the best that I know is located in the old downtown of Farmington, New Mexico, favored, like that long-ago Chinese restaurant in Tuba City, by a clientele of local Navajo families, along with workers from the nearby oil fields. Although there is anecdotal evidence to suggest that the first Thai restaurant can be traced to Denver, the first hard proof that we have dates only to 1968 and Los Angeles, where an entrepreneurial immigrant, Surabon Mekpongsatorn, opened several Thai restaurants in and near Alhambra, where a small Thai community had taken root to the east of the metropolitan area's existing Chinatown and Koreatown.

The United States does not have a lock on the market for interest in foreign cuisines. South Korea recently went through a donut craze. Lately, extending the globalism that has marked the economy of the last few generations, another craze has struck there, for young people in Korea are devouring—yes, tacos,

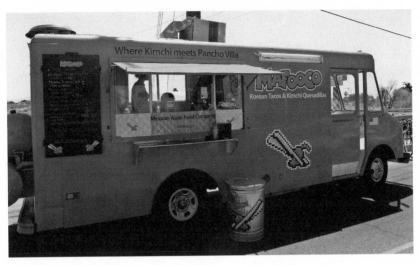

Korean and Mexican food traditions meet in a Tucson truck.

with the addition of pickled vegetables called kimchi to internationalize that ancient Aztec dish even more. It's fusion at its finest, a phenomenon that we have seen repeated with one food tradition after another in this country. Nowhere is that more evident than in the Los Angeles district called Korea-town, populated by successive waves of arrivals from the Korean Peninsula, beginning with a trickle a century ago and expanding with immigration reform in the mid-1960s.

One of the great success stories to emerge from there owes to an entrepreneur named Mark Manguera, who combined the fixings of a traditional Southwestern taco with Korean barbecue in 2008 and sent a young employee named Roy Choi out in a food truck to sell the concoction. Recalls Choi, who later became a celebrity chef,

> The Korean taco was a phenomenon. . . . It just came out of us, we didn't really think about it. The flavor, in a way, didn't exist before, but it was a mash up of everything we had gone through in our lives. It became a voice for a certain part of Los Angeles and a certain part of immigration and a certain part of life that wasn't really out there in the universe. We all knew it and we all grew up with it, and it was all around us, but the taco kind of pulled it together. It was like a lint roller; it just put

everything onto one thing. And then when you ate it, it all of a sudden made sense.

It certainly did, and after Kogi's, as the mobile restaurant was named, netted more than a million dollars in its first year of operation, other food vendors took notice. Korean fusion food has rapidly spread throughout Southern California and the rest of the Southwest. On my last visit to Austin's food trucks, it seemed that the Korean-themed trucks were doing the most business, though the lines were happily long for every kind of fare.

Los Angeles makes an interesting case study for an immigrant future that is likely to be reflected elsewhere in the Southwest. The three heaviest concentrations of Asian Americans in the United States are to be found there, in Los Angeles County, Santa Clara County, and Orange County, in that order. Irvine, the home of John Wayne International Airport, is 45 percent Asian and a lively food destination as a result, particularly, these days, for its Taiwanese bakeries, which offer squid-ink bread, pork-topped hot buns, and sweet rolls. The fastest-growing immigrant population in the city as I write is from Bangladesh, which likely means that soon Irvine will be home to restaurants representing the full range of foods from the country.

More so than most "world cities," Los Angeles really is a microcosm of the world, in which you are likely, if you look hard enough, to find one of every kind of person on the planet, every tribe and clan and nation. Parts of the city bear names such as Little Armenia, in Los Angeles, and Tehrangeles, the latter honoring the eight hundred thousand or so Iranians who live on the city's west side and in the San Fernando Valley, the largest population of Iranians outside Iran itself. With large populations of Filipinos, Chinese, Koreans, Burmese, Laotians, Cambodians, Afghans, South Asians, and so forth, the metropolis has seen a blossoming of a hundred kinds of restaurants. It would take decades to eat one's way through them. About the only form of Asian food that has never caught on in Los Angeles, or anywhere else in the Southwest, for that matter, is Mongolian barbecue, which enjoyed a brief fad in the 1990s but seemingly could not compete with the many forms of barbecued meat already on offer.

Writing in the *New York Times*, Nathaniel Rich celebrates this city of "miniature homelands" as a harbinger of an atomized future in which strangers would be welcome to visit for a meal, though likely not be made fully at home; he enumerates, "Little India, Little Russia, Koreatown, Japantown, half a million Iranians, Little Armenia, Little Osaka, Little Saigon, Filipino-town, and of course Chinatown." All that, of course, in addition to the neigh-borhoods made up of people from every Central and South American nation, every European country, just about every African land.

It is a strange thing that this California, the land of sunshine, oranges, the Beach Boys, and other signs and portents of optimism, should also have bred some of the darkest visions of the future known to science fiction, or, better, sci-fi—a term coined by California editor and novelist Forrest Ackerman in the 1950s. The Golden State's contributions to science fiction are many, and they are relentlessly gloomy, from the dystopian visions of Philip K. Dick to the dyspeptic scenarios of Harlan Ellison, the cryptofascist man-versus-insect dreams of Robert Heinlein, and the authoritarian shoot-'em-ups of Jerry Pournelle.

Even the comparatively kindhearted Ray Bradbury had his doubts about earthlings—as one might, caught in traffic with so many of them, which a few minutes on the 405 or the 101 will instruct you. Still, Rich finds hope in a future marked by class and ethnic division and all manner of strife. "If the future is *Blade Runner*," he writes, "then we'll have yummy noodles and hot sauce." It could be much worse.

10. **Corporatization and Standardization**

Consider the Caesar salad, a simple dish made elegant, in its classic form, by tableside preparation. The table in question was originally a single restaurant just across the international line from San Diego, California, the time the cheerless years of Prohibition, when an Italian-born restaurateur named Cesare Cardini moved his operations to Mexico so that he could keep serving alcohol with his meals. The origin story continues: On a particularly busy and bibulous holiday weekend in 1924, Cardini found that he was out of the usual ingredients for his insalata mista, and he rounded up what he could from nearby shops and his cupboards—romaine lettuce, parmesan cheese, lemons, bread cubes, olive oil, eggs, some Worcestershire sauce. Perhaps in pique but with grand flair and *bella figura*, Cardini had his chef toss the salad at the tables of those who ordered salad with their meal.

An iconic food thus made its way into the world, and by the 1940s the Caesar salad, so spelled, was a fixture at fine restaurants around the world—for Cardini did not attempt to patent his invention until decades after the fact. His Hotel Caesar became a foodie destination all the same, tourists convening there for a taste of the real thing at its birthplace, and Cardini—and then, after his death in 1956, his daughter Rosa and her family—enjoyed a brisk business.

All that ended in 2009, however, a dark year that saw horrific drug-related violence swallow up the Southwestern borderlands, the ceaseless appetite for drugs north of the border satisfied by monsters to the south. An unfortunately coincidental outbreak of avian flu, the deepest throes of the Great Recession in the United States, and the rise of appallingly ugly nativist xenophobia all conspired to halt the tourist trade into Mexico. It has yet to recover.

Caesar Salad

The salad that bears Cesare Cardini's name is now a world standard. Here is his original recipe.

3 heads romaine lettuce
1 cup olive oil
2 cloves garlic, peeled and crushed
⅓ baguette, cut crosswise into ¼-inch slices
Juice of 1 lemon
1 tablespoon red wine vinegar
Dash worcestershire sauce
1 egg, coddled for 1 minute
½ cup freshly grated parmigiano-reggiano cheese
Salt and freshly ground black pepper

Trim about 1 inch from the bottom of each head of lettuce and peel away all dark green leaves until you reach the pale-green-tipped yellow leaves, or heart of the lettuce (the longest leaves should be no longer than 7 inches). Discard outer leaves or save for another use. Separate leaves, wash, then pat dry thoroughly with paper towels; set aside.

Heat ⅔ cup of the oil with the garlic in a medium skillet over medium heat until garlic is golden, about 5 minutes, then remove and discard garlic. Fry bread slices in oil in batches until deep golden, 15–20 seconds per side. Use tongs or a slotted spoon to transfer croutons to a plate, and set aside.

Put lemon juice, vinegar, and worcestershire sauce in a large wooden salad bowl, crack coddled egg into bowl, and mix vigorously with a wooden spoon or spatula until smooth. Gradually add remaining ⅓ cup oil, stirring constantly. Add cheese and season to taste with salt and pepper. Add croutons, then lettuce, and toss well.

On September 28, 1914, a shopkeeper turned magnate drew his last breath. He was only fifty. But in the course of his half century, Richard Warren Sears made mercantile history, and he changed the face of American commerce, especially outside the nation's big cities.

When Sears was born, at the end of 1863, most Americans lived in small towns or on farms. They were supplied, with difficulty and at much expense, by a network of roads and railroads, and, in the hinterlands of the frontier, by freight wagons that were the equivalent of the toughest four-wheel-drive vehicles today. In return, they sent their goods, whether firearms or furniture or food, to other places by that same network. It became less unwieldy in time, however, owing to the vision of industrialists such as Andrew Carnegie and Leland Stanford, who saw the importance of transportation in uniting a far-flung nation—the very insight that drove Fred Harvey to develop his food empire in the wake of the infrastructure they built.

Then a railroad station manager on the Minnesota frontier, Sears had a chance bit of luck in 1886. A common practice of the time was for wholesalers to ship goods to merchants that they had not ordered but even so would often keep just to save the expense of sending them back—for that was well before the time of free return shipping. A local merchant, receiving such a shipment of unasked-for, expensive pocket watches, refused to accept them. Sears contacted the wholesaler and negotiated a low price for them, for the wholesaler didn't want to pay return freight either, and then he set about selling those watches to his fellow railroad workers, time being every bit of the essence to that audience.

Sears pocketed a profit of $5,000, or about $120,000 today, which he reckoned was enough starting capital to quit his railroad job and head for the big city of Minneapolis, where he established the R. W. Sears Watch Co. Ever an innovator, he considered how poor was the access his rural customers had to goods, and he inaugurated what might be considered business history's first targeted mailing campaign to advertise his goods.

The campaign worked, and Sears quickly transferred his operations to Chicago, then as now the most important transportation hub in the upper Midwest, with rail links nationwide. Soon after he arrived in Chicago, Sears took out an advertisement in a Chicago paper for a watch repairman. A newcomer from Indiana, Alvah Roebuck, replied and got the job.

Roebuck, who was a year younger than his partner, worked side by side with Sears for the next several years, eventually adding other products to the watch line: eyeglasses and other optical goods, jewelry, phonographs. In 1888 Sears began issuing a general catalog on top of his frequent mailers. The 1894 annual edition weighed in at 325 pages. If you lived in just about anywhere in the nation—from the Arctic Circle to the deepest canyons of the Navajo Nation—you could thumb through that catalog, pick out a product, enclose cash or a teller's check, and receive your good by return post. By 1895 the catalog was up to 530 pages, and by then you could buy rifles, canned goods, pocketknives, and irrigation pumps. By 1905 when the catalog was larger still, you could even buy an automobile or a kit to build a house.

The Sears Catalog, as it was known even before Roebuck left the partnership, was a critical ingredient in building the mail-order business of today, now dominated by Internet giants in just the way that Sears did in its time. What is more, it helped integrate consumer markets: You did not have to live in a big city to buy that pocketknife, of which the catalog had page after page, and there were no local variations—the Barlow knife was the Barlow knife from Apalachicola to Albuquerque and Atascadero.

A second ingredient in this integration came two years after Sears's death. In 1916 in the bustling river city of Memphis, Tennessee, the first completely self-service grocery store in America opened, the flagship of a chain that would become iconic in the South: Piggly Wiggly. Clarence Saunders, the store's owner, had put a great deal of thought into how his store would be laid out, and any would-be customers who wanted to come in and eventually get out had to make their way through a mazelike series of aisles that required them to see every single item the store had in stock. Out went the little shopping list, and in came eyes bigger than stomachs, overflowing cupboards, and the beginning of the modern era in American food consumption.

Clarence Saunders's innovation, clever if a touch heavy-handed, is not widely used these days. But there's a definite science behind how large grocery stores are laid out—a geography of the supermarket, so to speak. One of the key points of that geography is that the things we need the most—bread, milk, eggs, fresh vegetables, cheese, and meat—are located by design as far as they can be from the front door, forcing the shopper to navigate the entire store just as surely as if Saunders had laid out the path himself. The dairy section in particular is almost always at the farthest possible point away from the entrance. (If you are inclined toward what computer hackers call "social engineering," however, you can subvert this cunning plan by entering the store and then following a course around the outer walls, steering clear of the interior.)

There is a larger geography of food to acknowledge. In some parts of the country, notably the South and West, a certain kind of corn chip is highly popular. Travel to the mid-Atlantic region, and potato chips rise in popularity. Travel farther up the Atlantic coast, and brands of potato chips begin to show up that cannot be found in other parts of the country. Travel west from there and you'll find many more brands of salsa and tortillas than in an ordinary grocery in, say, New Hampshire. Travel back south and you'll find both Miracle Whip dressing and mayonnaise on the shelf, but likelier you'll find twice as many jars of the latter, since Southerners show a noted preference for mayonnaise and the foods with which it's eaten, such as potato salad and coleslaw. Hit the Potomac River and sweet tea disappears from the menu. Leave the upper Midwest and lutefisk can no longer be found.

Thanks to modern transportation systems and food preservatives, however, grocery stores show a remarkable sameness wherever you travel, even outside the country. One unavoidable facet is the shopping cart or trolley, invented in 1937, the brainchild of the manager of a Humpty Dumpty grocery store in Oklahoma who theorized that the more food a shopper could carry, the more she or he was likely to buy.

All of this has bearing on the experimentation, social and commercial, that grocers in Southern California have been conducting for years. Owing to broad affluence and ethically diverse communities alike, to say nothing of its car culture, the region has long been an incubator for grocery stores, with more than seven thousand outlets serving its huge population. One of the largest chains, Safeway, started in the 1920s but found its fortunes improved as it expanded in areas without strong local markets, which meant dusty desert towns in the interior. Other grocery chains followed, including Albertson's, Von's, and Lucky. A pioneer in the region's grocery business, Ralphs, was founded in 1879 near the heart of downtown Los Angeles. In 1926 following a disagreement with local bakeries over volume pricing, Ralphs established bakeries at its outlets, a custom that has since been emulated by nearly every major grocery chain. Though Ralphs still has hundreds of stores, it has never managed to capture a commanding market share, precisely because that competition is so fierce.

Trader Joe's, rapidly expanding nationwide, began life in the late 1950s as a neighborhood convenience store called Pronto Market, which went up against 7-Eleven, itself the brainchild of an employee at the Southland Ice Company of Dallas, Texas, who in 1927 began to sell bread, milk, and eggs on Sundays and at night, when regular groceries were closed. He named the impromptu store "Tote'm," then, in 1946, changed the name to 7-Eleven to mark his chain of stores' regular business hours. Joe Coulombe took the convenience store sideways, catering to customers with a taste for imported beers and wines and adding a deli counter to the mix. In 1979 Coulombe sold his chain, renamed Trader Joe's in apparent homage to the tiki-pioneer restaurant Trader Vic's, to the German supermarket magnate Theo Albrecht. Following Coulombe's retirement, the chain expanded out of California, first into neighboring Arizona and then other states.

Trader Joe's is now seen as a lower-priced competitor to the Texas giant Whole Foods, which began as an organic grocery in 1980 in Austin. In close competition with the Central Market spinoff of the H-E-B Grocery Company, Whole Foods has proven of critical importance in spreading "foodie" culture throughout the United States, and though it has been criticized on many counts, including high prices (not for nothing is it nicknamed "Whole Paycheck"), the chain has been one of the great success stories of the modern retail grocery business—a business with strong roots in the Southwest.

Asked to name her favorite snack food of a Super Bowl Sunday, Michelle Obama replied without hesitation, "Super Bowl food? You know, nachos are always good." Americans might be divided by politics, but they seem very much in favor of the first lady's gulf-bridging recommendation.

The nacho was born of a necessity that met with a bright stopgap measure. The story has it that during World War II a group of Army Air Corps pilots from a nearby Texas airfield crossed the border to Piedras Negras, Mexico, and after many a tipple made their way to El Moderno, a restaurant owned by a man named Ignacio Anaya. The kitchen had just closed, but Ignacio—a name affectionately shortened to "Nacho" in Mexican Spanish—whipped up a dish of reheated tortilla chips smothered with cheddar cheese instead of the usual queso blanco and sprinkled with chopped jalapeño peppers. Some accounts have the diners as the wives of Army officers and not the aviators themselves, but whoever ate Anaya's concoction, they left satisfied.

The Original Pantry in
Los Angeles, a twenty-
four-hour restaurant
whose doors have never
closed since 1929.

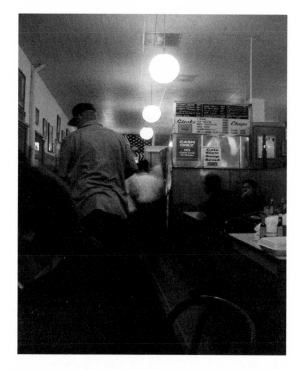

The resulting "nachos," as the new snack was called, wasn't an invention on the order of, say, the cotton gin or the polio vaccine, but it had its purpose, and the diners went off to spread the word, bringing El Moderno many new clients from across the line—a trade that prevailed until 2009, when El Moderno fell victim to the same forces that closed Caesar's in Tijuana.

How the nacho spread beyond that is a matter of historical mystery, though it is attested by that name as early as 1959 in Los Angeles. By the late 1970s nachos had become the snack of choice at the concession stands of the Texas Rangers stadium in Arlington. Given the team's lackluster history in the years since expansion landed the Rangers in the Dallas area, nachos have proved of more enduring popularity than the lineup. Remarked one stadium goer to sportswriter David McCollum, "Thinking about those nachos is better than thinking about the game."

Necessity is the mother of invention indeed. The corn chip, a close cousin of the nacho whose official birthdate precedes it by a couple of decades, first bowed in at a diner in San Antonio owned by a Mexican immigrant named

Gustavo Olguin. Olguin, it seems, was experimenting with something that crossed the consistency of the tortilla chip with the taste of the hush puppy. When, at the dawn of the Great Depression, he decided to return home, he sold an adapted potato ricer used to make the corn chips and the recipe for them to Charles Elmer Doolin, who worked at the diner as a fry cook. According to Kaleta Doolin, his daughter, Doolin further experimented in his family's bakery in Highland Park, improving on the recipe until he finally developed a chip that would not go stale as quickly as ordinary tortilla chips.

In 1932 Doolin took out a trademark on the name Frito, from the Spanish word for "fried." The same year Herman W. Lay of Nashville, Tennessee, began to sell a potato chip that met with instant success. The two entrepreneurs operated independently until, in 1945, their paths crossed, and Doolin granted Lay the right to sell his chips in the Southeast. The companies merged in September 1961, by which time Doolin had been growing fields of his own hybridized corn and from time to time adding products to his line, such as Cheetos, a kind of nacho reduced to essential form, at least if you are inclined to continental philosophy. Another addition came in 1964, when an executive of the recently founded Frito-Lay Company, vacationing in California, bought a bag of tortilla chips from a roadside stand. He divined that the heavily salted chip would make a fine mass-produced snack food to complement the company's signature Frito line, and so, borrowing from the Spanish word for golden, *dorado*, Arch West coined the trade name "Dorito" for the product that Frito-Lay introduced nationally in 1966.

Fritos has remained one of the most popular snack chips on the market for decades, and perhaps improbably, given the offense raised by the company's long-abandoned "Frito Bandito" character, it is as likely to turn up in Hispanic as Anglo lunchboxes. The same is true of "Frito pie," a concoction that probably originated in an Anglo household, a simple blend of Texas-style chili, cheese, onions, and Fritos. Born in Texas, it was popularized by Teresa Hernández, a server at Woolworth's on the plaza in Santa Fe, New Mexico, who sold thousands of Frito pies—more than fifty thousand in one year in the early 1960s—making use of her mother's altogether more robust chile rojo. Alas, the Frito pie has long since been tamed, and the chile is almost always back to being chili, and with beans to boot.

Coconut Cream Pie

Before he loaned his name to a mass-manufactured packaged cake mix that is another staple of American grocery stores, Duncan Hines (1880–1959) was one of the best-known restaurant critics in the United States. He crisscrossed the country, giving his seal of approval (or stern notes to the contrary) and collecting recipes. Here, with slight modifications, is one that he gathered from the Encanto Tea Shop in Los Angeles in about 1940.

1 cup milk
1 ⅓ cups sugar
Pinch of salt
2 egg yolks, beaten
2 tablespoons cornstarch
1 tablespoon milk
2 ½ teaspoons unflavored gelatin
1 tablespoon milk
½ cup coconut
1 cup whipped cream
1 teaspoon vanilla
2 egg whites, beaten
1 10-inch pastry shell (Graham cracker crust is best)

Combine the first three ingredients in a saucepan. Bring to a boil. Blend cornstarch and 1 tablespoon milk and mix with eggs. Add to hot milk above and cook slightly.

Dissolve gelatin in 1 tablespoon milk and pour hot mixture over it. Let set until firm. Put in electric beater and beat well.

Add coconut, whipped cream, and vanilla and refrigerate for 10 minutes. Fold in stiff egg whites; pour in baked pastry shell; cover with whipped cream and sprinkle with coconut.

The automobile came into widespread use in the United States in the early years of the twentieth century, and no place seemed more welcoming than the wide-open Southwest.

Automobiles hadn't been around long when, in 1903, a Tucson physician named H. W. Fenner decided to purchase a 1900 Locomobile steamer, a contraption that looked like little more than a buckboard wagon with a tiny engine, one that wheezed and banged just loud enough to frighten a horse. Dr. Fenner took quite a liking to driving through the dirt streets of downtown Tucson, tipping his hat and gladly receiving the looks of admiration that came his way.

He had the road to himself for a couple of years. By 1905, however, when Fenner was issued the first driver's license in the Arizona Territory, other moneyed Tucsonans had imported horseless carriages from eastern factories, and downtown windows soon rattled with traffic noise. "Old Doc" Fenner, who was all of forty, was happy to chug along at a snail's pace, but younger drivers needed a place to push their roadsters to the limit, which in those days was the daredevil speed of 15 miles per hour.

Tucson's constabulary quickly made it clear that downtown was no place to tear around in but seemed not to mind if the youngsters zoomed along any of the graded dirt roads that led out of the downtown area to points east and west. One such road, thanks to marvels of land velocity demonstrated by the likes of merchant Frank Steinfeld's 1911 Stutz Bearcat—it could get up to 20 miles per hour—soon bore the congratulatory name Speedway.

It's no accident that Speedway, soon thereafter and eleven decades later and all the time in between, should have been a locus for fast-food restaurants. But as for the origins of those revolutionary things, we need to look farther west, to California, where car culture really came into its own. The first of them sprang forth Athena-like from an entrepreneur in Lodi, California, named Roy Allen, who opened a root beer stand on June 20, 1919, that proved so successful that within a year he opened several other stands in Modesto, Stockton, Sacramento, and elsewhere in the Central Valley. To help manage his growing empire, he took on a partner named Frank Wright, and A&W Root Beer was born. In time, A&W stands, of which there were more than two hundred franchise outlets by the mid-1930s, began selling food—hamburgers, mostly, but in some Southern California locations tacos and other Mexican items.

The A&W model was well in the minds of the brothers Richard McDonald

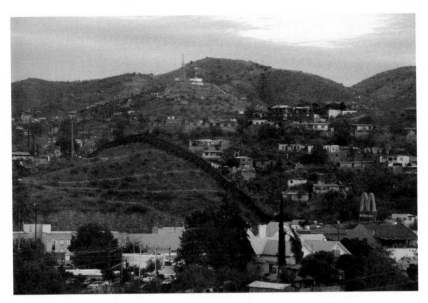

Nogales, Arizona: The border wall looms, but the golden arches call.

and Maurice McDonald, who opened a hot dog stand in Arcadia, California, in 1937, then sold it and moved east to San Bernardino, where they opened a barbecue restaurant. Dick and Mac were shrewd, analytically minded businessmen, and they soon determined that hamburgers were more profitable than the other items on their menu, on account of which they closed their doors and reopened as a walk-up hamburger stand. They did so well along postwar Route 66 that they experimented with franchising their menu and licensing the design of their San Bernardino flagship, whose overhanging roof now bore supporting yellow arches. When a milkshake machine salesman named Ray Kroc came calling in 1954, history was made: Kroc bought the original restaurant and its franchise rights in 1955, launching another food empire.

Wisely, recognizing that McDonalds sounded better than Kroc's, he kept the original name. It's one of the curiosities of history, by the way, that Walt Disney and Ray Kroc served together in an ambulance unit in World War I. Kroc spent his leisure time in French restaurants, while Disney carefully shot holes in discarded German helmets, painted them with chicken blood, and then sold them to his fellow soldiers. Disney's arts of deception would soon alter the very landscape of California, though Kroc seems to have kept his knowledge of haute cuisine to himself. These details, by the way, are from a third ambulance man in that unit, Waverley Root, who would go on to write pioneering books of food history.

The year 1948 saw the birth of another iconic Southwestern hamburger chain, far distant from McDonald's Famous Hamburgers in San Bernardino but right next door to the McDonalds' first stand, at least as distances in Southern California go. Esther and Harry Snyder worked from an elegantly simple business model: They would not use the newfangled invention called the heat lamp or the steam table in their restaurant but would instead cook hamburgers fresh and to order and would serve them with fresh vegetables. Their In-N-Out Drive-In in Baldwin Park was an immediate hit, but, unlike Ray Kroc, they were slow to build on it; thirty years later, they had only a dozen and a half locations scattered throughout metropolitan Los Angeles, and these were the stuff of legend, frequented by rock stars and movie actors as well as beach bums and knowing tourists. In-N-Out has since expanded, though fans still think of it as their secret. I'm one of those fans, and though In-N-Out is now all over Arizona (and the I-35 corridor of Texas, though not yet in New Mexico), I still prefer to partake west of the Colorado River, that strategy being better for my waistline than otherwise. In-N-Out has the distinction of being fast food that is seen, for many reasons, as better than fast food, and it has served as the model for many other chains, such as Blake's Lotaburger—which *is* all over New Mexico, headquartered in Albuquerque and so famed for its green chile burger that it has recently opened locations in El Paso and Tucson.

In 1951 a California restaurateur named Glen Bell decided to branch out, selling crispy-shell tacos at nineteen cents apiece from his San Bernardino emporium. He had borrowed liberally from a more formal restaurant across the street, the Mitla Cafe, which had been doing a steady trade since opening in 1937, making it the oldest Mexican restaurant in the so-called Inland Empire, which scarcely existed before the postwar boom. So successful was he that over the next decade, Bell's Hamburgers and Hot Dogs spawned several restaurants in Southern California, including three in the El Taco chain. In 1962 these were unified under the Taco Bell name. By 1978 when he sold the brand to PepsiCo, Bell's empire had grown to 868 shops; there are about 5,600 Taco Bell restaurants today.

Though it might pain an aficionado of authentic cuisine to admit it, Glen

Bell's Taco Bell has been perhaps the single greatest force in spreading the taco as we know it—not tlacoyo, not tamale, but the familiar flat, fried, meat-filled taco—beyond the Southwest and out into the hungry world. But two other Anglo vendors deserve some credit for that work as well.

The first, whose history goes back to 1927, was a decided outlier. Willard Marriott and his wife, Alice, who hailed from ranching families in Utah and had traveled throughout the Southwest, moved to Washington, DC, and that year opened a diner selling tamales and chile. There were a few other places in the capital that served Mexican food to homesick Southwesterners, but Hot Shoppes soon became a local favorite, even though tamales and chile were crowded out by fried chicken and Big Boy hamburgers.

The second was a Texan named Louis Stumberg, whose family had been in the food business ever since opening up a market within sight of the Alamo in 1846. There they took their place in a thriving industry that, beginning in the 1870s, saw the commodification of Mexican food products such as canned chile sauce and dried chile powder, which enjoyed large markets in African American communities in the Midwest, the very place where tamales were popular. Entrepreneur William Gebhardt, for instance, sold chili as well as German food at his restaurant in New Braunfels, selling chile powder first as "Tampico Dust" and then under the more genteel name of Gebhardt's Eagle Brand Chili Powder. Other Texas vendors made a hit of "San Antonio chili" at the Columbian Exposition in Chicago in 1893, building an audience for Mexican food outside the city's already large Mexican population.

But it was not until the immediate aftermath of World War II that various ingredients came together. Stumberg was working in a thankless job selling frozen vegetables to markets in West Texas. Facing stiff competition from national suppliers, he had the inspired thought that the military bases in which Texas abounded might make a ready market for already made meals featuring popular Tex-Mex dishes such as chile con carne as well as tamales, enchiladas, burritos, and refried beans. Stumberg's Patio Foods, founded in San Antonio, took that cuisine nationwide in the late 1950s, a pioneer in the Mexican TV dinners that populate the memories of just about any American, I'd warrant, who was conscious and cognizant in the 1960s, and a meal of choice to eat while watching *Daniel Boone*.

Grocery stores, cars, fast food. A critical ingredient in bringing all these things to the fore nationwide were the technological and social revolutions wrought by World War II, the memory of which was fresh to the point of rawness in the dawning age of the TV dinner. For the first time in the nation's history, that conflict brought technicians, scientists, businessmen, politicians, civil servants, teachers, and craftsmen together into a common cause, for earlier wars were fought mostly by farm boys and the urban poor. The mixing of their ideas produced a technological revolution that buoyed the economy of the postwar world and placed America in the vanguard of global commerce. It also laid the Great Depression to rest once and for all, yielding a new prosperity and the rise of the consumer culture.

Some of those technological changes are obvious. The mushroom cloud following our use of atomic weapons against Japan, for instance, helps define our image of the postwar world. Less well known are the many changes in our lives that came about when military technology was converted to civilian use, from nuclear power plants to the popular meat product called Spam.

The American housewife—as a stay-at-home woman of the time was called—of the 1940s and '50s was one of the earliest beneficiaries of this shift in production. Developed for use in military hospitals, for instance, electric clothes dryers came out on the civilian market just a year after V-J Day. By the end of the decade they were selling by the thousands, along with garbage disposals and automatic dishwashers, once giant machines miniaturized for portability during the war.

Other such machines were the home refrigerator and freezer. During the war, the need to ship and store food in difficult conditions led to many changes in refrigeration technology. Inexpensive home-size refrigerators came about when military planners found they needed to cool military aircraft engines flying over long distances. They hit upon the small compressor—the unit at the back of your home box—as a ready solution, and the kitchen fridge was born. It became a great postwar success: in 1930, only twenty-five thousand American households boasted iceboxes, but there are now more than 125 million of them in the United States. That path of growth has been replicated worldwide, and when I interviewed her a few years ago, the British food writer Bee Wilson pointed out that the refrigerator "has taken over from fire as the focus around which our kitchens are built. Its importance goes far beyond cooking."

Another wartime invention took nearly three decades to become common in American homes. This was the microwave oven, first developed in the mid-1940s in order to shape magnetrons for military radars. In 1946 an engineer at the then-tiny Raytheon Corporation in Boston—later to relocate to Tucson—a man notorious for his sweet tooth, happened to be standing in front of an oven while conducting experiments. When a candy bar in his pocket instantly melted, he realized that the oven could be used to cook food—and at a considerable savings in energy over conventional ovens. By 1952 the engineer had secured a patent for a commercial microwave oven. The prototype stood over six feet tall. It took a generation of tinkerers two more decades to shrink the microwave down to countertop size.

No matter how dreary their lives might become, postwar housewives had a far easier time than their prewar peers. In the 1930s America was still a rural nation, and at the beginning of that decade only 13 percent of all farms had electricity. On average, farmwomen had to haul thirty tons of water by hand every year from wells or springs into their homes; indoor plumbing was equally scarce. The advent of World War II launched federal programs to electrify and mechanize rural America. Only at the end of the war were most combines machine-powered. Only at the end of the war were pesticides—most, like DDT, invented for military use—heavily used. Most significantly, almost a third of the farmland in the United States today was put into production during the war.

Mechanization was successful enough that by 1960 only 3 percent of America's people still farmed. Most of the rest of us lived in cities or in another postwar invention: the suburb. But one nearly universal item in the American repertoire today was worn on farms and in cities and suburbs alike: blue jeans. Invented by the itinerant Jewish tailor Levi Strauss for miners during the California Gold Rush of 1849, these durable trousers clothed millions of American sailors during World War II. When the tars came home, their pants came with them, and by the early 1950s jeans were clothing millions of civilians. The next time you see the film *The Wild One*, count the number of jeans wearers among the good guys and bad guys alike: If there were ever an American shibboleth, it was not clad in denim.

Battle brought together technicians, scientists, businessmen, politicians, civil servants, teachers, and craftsmen, all right. But it also brought together New Englander and Southerner, Easterner and Westerner, Hispano and African American and Native American and Anglo. They fought together. They also ate together, exchanging fond memories of local foods that would become wider spread after the war—tamales in Bangor, bagels in Phoenix, tortilla chips in Honolulu.

American tastes changed considerably in those postwar years. Intensive industrial farming methods changed the face of the livestock industry once again, boosting production to meet the demands of a market grown prosperous. Refrigeration and transportation brought those meats and other goods nationwide so that markets were able to offer foods out of season. Thanks to those technological changes, the entire chain of food supply in the United States was transformed so that, for the first time in history, fresh vegetables, fresh meat, and fresh milk were available to consumers year-round. The effects were immediate. For one thing, American consumption of beef skyrocketed after World War II, peaking in 1979 at nearly 90 pounds per person annually. Per capita consumption of chicken tripled between the end of World War II and 2010. Pork consumption has grown less markedly, but it has grown all the same. No food item except fish, on a per-capita basis, has declined during the postwar era.

Production and consumption: All these changes are the fruits of standardization and corporatization, the very forces that took the Caesar salad from its modest birthplace in Tijuana to the head of the table worldwide.

II. Drink

The different regions of the Southwest have their characteristic plants: the saguaro of the Sonoran Desert, the cedar of the Texas Hill Country, the madrone of the California coast. Broadly distributed throughout the region, the agave, a member of the lily family often confused for a kind of cactus, is perhaps the most characteristic plant of the Southwest as a whole. The American varieties, long-ago immigrants from the rainforest of Central America, are particularly abundant in the Chihuahuan Desert, which occupies much of northern Mexico, New Mexico, and Texas, and they grow as well in the neighboring deserts of Arizona and California. There they were great gifts to the indigenous peoples of those regions, who used the heart of the plant for food, the spines for sewing needles and fishhooks, the spidery fibers of the fat leaves for fiber, and the sap for tangy drinks such as pulque and tiswin. And not just humans, but also many other animals— such as bats, moths, bees, hummingbirds, javelina, and coyotes— delight in a nectar that is dankly sweet when new, hinting at the taste of the liquid that can be conjured from within.

Throughout the Southwest, Native peoples gathered agaves just before flowering, when their sugars were concentrated at their peak, and slow-roasted the hearts. The labor required was intensive, for first the agave had to be uprooted, and then the

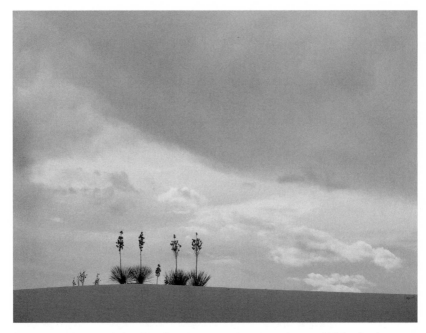

Agaves are characteristic of the Southwestern deserts, as here at White Sands National Monument, New Mexico.

spiky leaves, or *pencas*, had to be cleared away, not an easy task with stone tools and still a workout today using a steel machete. A large plant can have a heart weighing from fifty to as much as a hundred pounds, and this would have had to be carried off to the encampment and campfires of the people doing the gathering. The hearts were typically roasted in fire pits covered with branches or stones, in much the manner of a pig cooked at a luau, a process that took days as the starches converted to sugars that could then be extracted in edible form.

The work was great, but the payoff was substantial, and for that reason a hallmark of many prehistoric settlements was the agave roasting pit. Moreover, many prehistoric settlements in the Southwest became agave cultivation hubs. Hohokam villages along the Santa Cruz River in present-day Tucson, for example, were surrounded by fields of agaves numbering in the thousands, very much like the hills around Tequila, Mexico, are the site of spokes of agaves radiating from the hub of the town. Some species of agave cultivated in the desert, it is believed, were imported from deep within Mexico; as archaeologists Suzanne Fish and her colleagues carefully observe, "as with most other Southwestern aboriginal crops, cultivars may have included varieties of ultimate Mesoamerican origin."

Similarly, the eminent botanist Howard Scott Gentry noted,

> In Mesoamerica the many evolving varieties and forms of agave species were selected by man, moved from place to place with him, and inadvertently crossed. As man lived with these varietal eventualities through the centuries, he was provided with new genetic combinations that he could check empirically for yield and quality of fiber, food, beverage, and other special products. As he specialized with civilization, he specialized agave, selecting characteristics according to his wants. Even though he had no concept of genetics, he quite innocently fostered an explosive evolution in agave diversification.

In the Southwest these plants were doubtless prized for properties that included their ability to live in arid conditions—to say nothing of their ability to pack a punch.

Long ago some Native mescalero, or maker of mescal, perfected a means of extracting liquor from the liquid-filled hearts of the agave using fire and time. Tequila, bacanora, pulque, mescal, and other drinks of varying strengths and flavors resulted. Pulque likely came first, for it is the simplest of the alcoholic drinks to be made from agave, created before the introduction of distillation from Europe. It is traditionally made by sapping the plant's sugar-filled liquid, called *aguamiel*, or "honey water," into hollows carved in the heart and fermenting it into a milky drink about as strong as wine, about 10 percent alcohol. Pulque is decidedly inebriating, but, like beer, it is also a form of nutrition, packed with vegetable protein. All agaves produce sap from which aguamiel can be made, and the technology for making pulque was simple, making it among the most popular drinks in prehistoric Mesoamerica and the Southwest. Pulque has lost much of its popularity in recent times in Mexico, displaced by soft drinks and beer, but it is enjoying a modest revival as an artisanal product there, just as in recent years, Native peoples including the Mescalero, or agave-harvesting, Apaches of New Mexico and the Yavapai of Arizona have revived agave roasting traditions, even as ethnobotanists have identified new species of agaves that they and their neighbors used.

Mescal is a more complex distillate, probably first made after the arrival of the Spanish. In Sonora, a prized variant, made from *Agave anguistifolia*, is often concocted on ranches and in small towns in artisanal batches. On occasion, bottles, mason jars, plastic soda bottles, and milk jugs of this bacanora make their way across the border. A Southwestern version of white lightning, it is now being made commercially in Sonora after having been legalized in 1992, and specialty liquor stores across the border sometimes carry it. In the same way, sotol, made from agave's cousin Dasylirion, comes from neighboring Chihuahua, the Mexican state bordering westernmost Texas and New Mexico; connoisseurs prize sotol for its rich flavor.

By far the best-known agave distillate on this side of the international line is tequila, whose origins lie in the west-central Mexican state of Jalisco. Tequila has been made in commercial quantities since the mid-1800s there, with about half of its output since that time exported to the United States, and especially the Southwest, where it long ago worked its way into popular drinks such as the tequila sunrise and the margarita. The latter hails from the state of Jalisco and dates only to the 1920s, though something like it surely existed before then. A restaurateur in the capital city of Guadalajara, it's said, was idling a quiet afternoon away drinking a little tequila and nibbling on a blood orange half on which he'd sprinkled salt and chile powder. The taste combination proved pleasing, and the margarita soon became a signature drink at the restaurant, called La Viuda in some accounts and Los Sanchez in others. The drink soon became popular throughout the region, then Mexico, and then the Southwest, and now is a staple of bars the world over.

Tequila was a favorite item for smuggling across the border during the years of Prohibition, when thirsty Southwesterners drank it as never before. Throughout the 1940s and 1950s, it was periodically rediscovered as the preferred drink of hipsters, enshrined in the Champs' 1958 hit song "Tequila," enshrined anew in the Eagles' 1972 hit "Tequila Sunrise," a song that for a time distilled everything that was Southwestern in a few well-deployed chords.

So well established was the industry that when I lived in Guadalajara in the early 1980s, a handful of manufacturers dominated the market, and most

Margarita

My friend Richard Dooley, scion of an old Arizona family and inventor of the delicious and time-saving Dick's Mix margarita mix, serves a mean drink. Here is his recipe for the Mexican classic called the margarita, given a Southwestern twist.

GLASS PREPARATION
Avoid stemware of any kind. A 6–10 ounce glass is recommended because, should a guest not want to finish his or her drink, less is wasted.

At least 2 hours before serving, take a lime wedge and run it along only half of the rim of the glass. Press this half into a shallow layer of kosher salt on a saucer. Tap the glass so that any extra salt falls back onto the saucer.

The purpose of pre-salting a glass is so that by the time the drink is served, the salt has dried and stays adhered to the rim and it will take a few sips before it starts to loosen.

Salting only half the glass eliminates having to ask your guest if they want salt or not.

MARGARITA
In a blender, add:
5 ounces of premium orange liqueur (not triple sec!)
7 ounces of 100 percent agave tequila (silver or reposado)
4 ½ ounces of fresh-squeezed lime juice
2 ounces agave nectar
1 ounce raw sugar or honey

Add ice. Blend. Pour. Imbibe. Enjoy. Repeat if desired.

As to the Southwestern twist, Richard recommends adding prickly pear: Pick 4–6 tunas (prickly pear fruits). Wash thoroughly. Juice. Strain the juice with a fine strainer and even cheesecloth if available. Add only 2 ounces of the lime juice above and 4 ounces of prickly pear.

younger Mexicans seemed to think of tequila as an old-fashioned drink that their grandparents produced on special occasions, something that was part of their country's culinary heritage but not so very hip. Not so today. The blue agave, from which tequila (and agave nectar, another product growing in popularity) is made, represents the most intensively cultivated of the two hundred or so agave species found in Mexico and the desert Southwest, and the drink—known formally until recent times as "mescal wine from Tequila"—has since become subject to the same market forces as other controlled-origin drinks around the world, with true tequila coming only from the town in Jalisco that is its namesake, as well as a few authorized satellite distilleries in the neighboring states of Nayarit, Michoacán, and Guanajuato, along with a few in the noncontiguous Gulf Coast state of Tamaulipas.

Since 2000, a revival of interest in agave-based drink has led to an explosion in output and in artisanal production, with some 760 brands of tequila produced within Mexico and another 250 or so authorized for bulk export. Mescal (also spelled mezcal) has similarly enjoyed a great boom in popularity, made in small batches but now also produced by the distillery giant Bacardi, which makes it in a factory capable of but not yet producing 4.5 million liters a year. The largest tequila brands, foremost among them Cuervo and Sauza, still dominate the $2 billion market, but in recent years, manufacturers have begun to market a dizzying variety of oak-barrel-aged añejo and reposado varieties, a sampling of which I enjoyed several years ago with Rick Bayless and a colleague of his who, for want of a better term, might be called a tequila sommelier, serving up *traguitos* of tequila that resembled fine wine as well as others with the more forthright fire of liquor—but always with the taste of the delicious, slightly acrid sap from which it originated.

Because agaves grow so abundantly in the wild in the Southwest, they are a favorite of regional gardens as well. *Agave mapisaga*, the source of pulque, is particularly graceful, a huge plant that, fortunately for growers, has fairly gentle "teeth" on its leaves, though the spikes at the end of its leaves can still poke a good hole in a person. In the United States it grows best in California and Arizona, where it can grow to a fifteen-foot diameter, so it requires some forethought to site the plant and decide what to plant around it. The blue agave, *Agave tequilana*, the source of tequila, can be a little fussier, but once established, it holds to a middling size and, because of its striking blue-green color, makes a wonderful color complement to flowers of various colors and shapes and to lighter-hued cacti as well.

Most common agaves are monocarpic, meaning they flower only once— and when they do, it's curtains for the parent plant. Not long ago, one octopus agave, a *vilmoriniana* in our collection that had been growing quietly and contentedly in our front garden for years, suddenly showed its kinship with that vegetable by sending forth a shoot that resembled a giant asparagus—so large that in the end it measured twenty-two feet in height. The weight of the flower stalk was eventually so great that the host plant toppled over in a heavy windstorm, a sad end to a long and happy life.

But not an end, after all, for beneath the dead agave, which was so big and heavy that I had to take a chainsaw to it in order to be able to clear it away section by section, stood a dozen pups that flourished under its leaves and had now taken root on their own. And so, the agave's cycle of life continues on through these clones, bringing beauty and splendor to a desert garden and, in so many ways, to desert lives.

In 1767 the chemist, inventor, and natural philosopher Joseph Priestley moved into an old house alongside a brewery in northern England. While he repaired his new quarters, he experimented with what was called "fixed air," a gas produced by the fermentation process in brewing, and in time discovered that it could be introduced into water to make an inexpensive substitute for natural mineral water. His oddly influential pamphlet *Impregnating Water with Fixed Air*, published in 1772, found a ready audience among fellow Enlightenment enthusiasts in America, including Benjamin Franklin and Thomas Jefferson, who saw in Priestley's experiments an advance in purifying public water supplies.

It wasn't long before entrepreneurs were commercializing the science, too. In 1810 a patent was issued to an American brewery to produce "imitation mineral water" using Priestley's method. In the 1830s southern brewers began to introduce herbs and spices to the formula, making "physicks," drinks mostly marketed for their medicinal purposes. From popular medicine to popular culture was an easy step, and by the 1870s root beer and its variants were being sold throughout the country. Nowhere were these drinks more popular than in the hot South and Southwest, and it is no accident that two of the most popular soda pop brands sold in the United States today had their origins there. The first is Coca-Cola, born in Atlanta in 1886—a year, as it happens, after the other was invented in Waco, Texas.

There, a young pharmacist named Charles Alderton spent his days compounding medicines for a stream of patients and then whipping up tonics at the pharmacy's soda fountain. A born experimenter with dozens of notebooks recording his experiments in mixology, Alderton hit on the formula for a particularly bracing drink in about 1885, when he began to serve the nameless beverage, a blend of root beer with bitters, pepsin, and spices, including chile. Locals called the drink, sold at the downtown Old Corner Drug Store, a "Waco," but when W. B. Morrison, the store's owner, took out a patent on the drink on December 1, 1885, he did so under the trade name "Dr. Pepper."

Numerous theories have been advanced about that name, but suffice it to say that the drink's peppery flavor remains its hallmark, even as Dr Pepper (now without the period) has become an internationally marketed brand. Less successful was another Waco innovation, Sun Tang Red Cream Soda, another brainchild of two chemists who concocted it in 1937. Sun Tang Red was locally known as "Big Red," and so it is known now, sold nationally but with its largest market in the belt along Interstate 35 from Dallas to San Antonio.

A final soft drink story figures in all this. In 1911 yet another chemist, Neil Ward, developed a recipe for a Priestley-descended flavored mineral water making use of orange zest and juice. He called his drink Orange Crush, perfecting his recipe in 1815. The following year, in Los Angeles, Ward partnered with a soft-drink bottler named Clayton Howel to market the drink, which Howel generously renamed Ward's Orange Crush. Howel improved on Ward's recipe a touch, though, by adding orange pulp to the drink, giving

---

Jamaica

Made of dried hibiscus calyxes soaked in water, jamaica is a favorite drink of Mexican communities along the border.

Bring 6 cups water to a boil. Stir in 1 cup sugar and allow to dissolve. Add a squeeze of honey. Add 2 cups dried hibiscus flowers (available in Mexican and Caribbean markets) and a stick or two of cinnamon, preferably true cinnamon and not cassia. Allow to cool, then strain out solids and serve over ice.

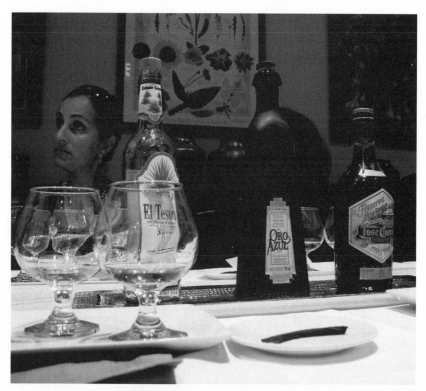

A tequila tasting at Frontera Grill, Rick Bayless's famed Chicago restaurant.

the illusion that the drink was made of freshly squeezed orange juice. Pulp has not been present in Orange Crush for many years, but the soft drink has become popular far outside its birthplace among the orange groves of Southern California.

Agave-based beverages were not the only alcoholic drinks that Native peoples of the Southwest consumed. With the arrival of corn, all those thousands of years ago, came a drink called tejuino in southern Mexico, tiswin or some variant thereof in several languages spoken in the borderlands country. Tiswin, made of boiled corn, water, and sometimes a sweetener such as honey that are blended and then fermented for several weeks, is a very lightly alcoholic drink. Often associated with religious ceremonies like Easter, it was usually made by women, whose involvement invested tiswin with significance and power. When Anglos arrived in the Southwest and established Indian reservations, they moved quickly to ban the use of tiswin on the grounds that it promoted drunkenness and lawlessness.

That was a misperception, though. Victor Randall, a Mescalero Apache, told the historian Eve Ball, who had asked him about tiswin binges, "A tiswin drunk? It wasn't tiswin that usually caused the trouble. We didn't have enough corn to make tiswin. It is not distilled; it's just fermented and about as strong as beer. It takes a lot of drinking to get drunk on tiswin. When you read about these tiswin drunks, just remember that they were mostly whiskey or tequila drunks."

Whiskey and tequila drunks would take their toll on Indian communities throughout the region, for decade on decade. But the Anglos were hardly in a position to be judgmental. In the early nineteenth century, at the stirrings of the era of westward expansion, Americans annually drank seven gallons of pure alcohol per capita, distributed in the form of various spirits. In terms of pure equivalence, that adds up to about two thousand 12-ounce cans of beer, or a little more than five and a half cans of beer each and every day of the week—but that figure does not even count the beer that was drunk in that time, consumed throughout the day as a mildly alcoholic safe form of drinking water, certainly safer than what came out of many public taps and wells in that day.

All that alcohol wrought its own damage, a constant companion of discord of all kinds, a ticket to violence, crime, and imprisonment. But as it had since the dawn of agriculture, beer was reckoned to be both a drink and a form of nourishment—a slice of bread in every glass, as the old saying goes—and the fact that beer was considered to play a fundamental part in the American diet placed a major obstacle in the way of teetotal campaigners in the second quarter of that century, men like William Lloyd Garrison, who, before gaining fame as an abolitionist, was an early champion of prohibition.

Garrison and his like-minded peers were considered oddballs. Like pioneer vegetarians, early teetotalers were thought to be suspect, even charged more in life insurance than drinkers because obviously somehow secretly ill. Even in the days of the frontier reformer Carrie Nation and the temperance movement, nondrinkers were a minority—and this was especially true of the Southwest, where whiskey, as it's said, was for drinking and water was for fighting over.

True, the "drys" had plenty of object lessons to hold up. One of the most eloquent of them was a fellow named George Hand, who left his native New York to go west to the gold fields of California in 1848. Having failed to make his fortune, he joined the Army and saw service in western Arizona and New Mexico during the Civil War, then made his way to Tucson and worked a variety of jobs—veterinarian, butcher, janitor, handyman—before opening a bar across the street from the courthouse. Hand drank up most of his proceeds, it seems, and spent the rest on prostitutes, but when he was not otherwise engaged he kept a diary of his life as a saloonkeeper, a diary that sheds fascinating light on frontier life in the 1870s and '80s. Here are a few passages:

Bedford was drunk all day—he talked several men nearly to death.

I took a bath, changed clothes, and feel tip-top for one who has been drunk for 6 years.

A new law firm has been established—Clark & McDermott. Principal business—drinking whiskey.

I went to bed at 9:30—slept very little—the streets were full of barking dogs and drunken whores.

Got drunk today. A Mexican cart ran over my little dog and killed him— had the funeral after dark. Shut the doors and two men had a fight.

Bob Morrow and Sherman came. Both got drunk, of course, I along with them. John Day got drunk—I found him in the church plaza.

Rainy and cloudy. Stage arrived—received a letter from Idaho. I got very drunk today. Dixon came in from Prescott, broke and sick.

There is great excitement about mines. Troy is drunk. He sold his blankets to bail old man Crosby out of jail and got drunk on the money.

Very warm day. Several drunken men were about. We had a light rain today. Closed at 11 o'clock.

Though Hand was unusually devoted to his drinking, which eventually killed him in 1887, he was by no means alone—and there was no shortage of things to drink about, since life in that dusty desert town had a certain Hobbesian quality to it. Violence was a daily affair, scarcely worth commenting over, though Hand's diary is full of casual references to it. Here are a few entries for the early fall of 1882:

> Fine morning. Two men dead. One natural death, the other named Hewitt, beaten until he died.

> Man killed last night.

> Chinaman got a bad beating this morning.

The following March, Wyatt Earp, then a deputy US Marshal, shot a man repeatedly at the train depot, which caused Hand to remark laconically, "Worst shot up man I ever saw." More seriously, he noted of a smallpox epidemic, "People formed a procession and marched from the church, singing and praying to the Patron Saint to stay the ravages of the fever now killing children every day."

Whiskey was relatively inexpensive in the East—a gallon cost twenty cents in 1852, about $40 today. Out on the frontier, the price would climb to two or three dollars for a bottle. Wrote one traveler to her family back home in the East, "That seems like a high price for liquor, but these men have to haul it from the States or from California, over the mountains, across the Great desert . . . so you see it is bound to be a costly drink."

That cost, as George Hand might have attested, did nothing to curb demand for drink. In Texas, men and women started the day with a mint julep first thing in the morning as "a healthful way to combat fevers, arising from night air and hot climates," as one Texan approvingly noted. Introduced by immigrant Kentuckians, the julep was widely considered a medicine more than a drink, a categorization that, as one might expect, can excuse any number of sins.

On the early frontier beer was less common than distilled spirits as a commercial product, in part because weak variants, the equivalents of tiswin, were made at home, top-fermented and drunk more or less fresh. American beer gained in both strength and popularity in the 1840s and especially after the Civil War, when an influx of immigrants from German-speaking countries, and later from points farther east in Europe, began to arrive in the Southwest in number. These newcomers drank lots of beer, and it is no accident that their arrival and their beer-drinking ways coincided with the first stirrings of the temperance movement that would eventually introduce Prohibition to the United States, an anti-immigrant and religious movement disguised as a public health campaign.

An epicenter of German immigration, Texas was also a hub for beer production in the Southwest, augmented by beer brewed in Mexico by German immigrants there and sold along the Arizona and New Mexico borderlands. Texas breweries specialized then as now in lager beer. The first to produce it in commercial quantities, William Menger's Western Brewery in San Antonio, flourished until 1878, when it closed, supplanted by competitors following the death of its master brewer—though before that time, it was producing sixteen hundred barrels of beer a year. In 1884 St. Louis brewer Adolphus Busch opened a factory in San Antonio that soon bore the name Lone Star. Within a couple of years, it was selling railroad-transported beer as far west as Los Angeles and deep into Mexico. Prohibition put an end to the original Lone Star, although another brewery assumed that name in 1940.

By 1900 Texas sported several dozen breweries that produced beer of superior strength and quality, enabling them to dominate the market throughout the larger region. They had some competition from breweries in northern California, such as Anchor in San Francisco, maker of the still-popular Anchor Steam beer and later a powerhouse of innovation for drinks ranging from wines to rye whiskey. For their part, brewers elsewhere in the Southwest did their best to meet local demand and compete with the Texas houses. In Tucson a Jewish immigrant named Alexander Levin established the first brewery in Arizona Territory in 1864, a boon for a population that included a substantial military garrison. Levin had honed his craft working in a German brewery in La Paz, on the tip of Mexico's Baja California peninsula, and would rank as a master brewer by any measure today, though in the end he abandoned brewing and went into the retail bar business, which did not suit him. In the meantime other breweries had sprung up elsewhere

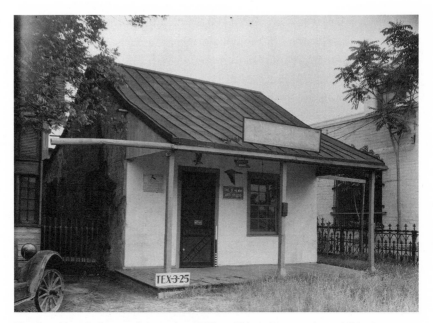

The San Antonio home of the writer William Sidney Porter, who published as O. Henry, once stood on the grounds of the Lone Star Brewery—an unfortunate convenience, given Porter's fatal fondness for drink. Courtesy of the Library of Congress.

in the territory, several in the mining centers of Bisbee and Tombstone and most associated with retail outlets.

That linkage has been revived in the last couple of decades in the microbrewery and brew pub industries, yielding fine beers from the Sonora Brewing Company of Phoenix, the Celis Brewery of Austin, the Little Toad Brewery in Silver City, and hundreds of others. Joining them were small-batch distillers across the region, offering vodka from Dripping Springs, whiskey from Bakersfield, absinthe from Santa Fe, and much more.

There has also been an explosion of craft wine production in every corner of the Southwest. The seeds of the wine industry, so to speak, were planted when the Spanish colonized the Rio Grande Valley in what is now New Mexico in the 1500s, planting vineyards along the fertile bottomlands. Spanish missionaries introduced wine production into Arizona and Texas as well, though it was the arrival of wine-loving German and Central European immigrants in the nineteenth century that revived production following the end of Spanish and Mexican rule in the latter. Among the earliest of them was the Val Verde vineyard of Del Rio, which has been in operation since 1833, though El Paso boasts the first vineyard in the state, thanks to the green-thumbed Fray García de San Francisco, whom we met earlier.

No state in the Southwest, though, has so strong an association with wine as California. In 1769 the Franciscan missionary Junípero Serra established a mission in what is now San Diego, and a decade later a vineyard was producing grapes sufficient for sacramental purposes and a little more. Wine production was connected to Spanish missions and other establishments of the Catholic Church for the first few decades of California settlement, with individual settlers, themselves mostly Catholic, planting small vineyards in new towns such as Los Angeles and Santa Barbara. A French immigrant named Jean-Louis Vignes was the first commercial grower in California, planting more than a hundred acres along the Los Angeles River and, by 1849, producing more than 150,000 bottles of wine yearly. Later arrivals set their mark on California winemaking, large and small. Wherever there was an Italian household, it was said, there was a vine; so widespread was home production of wine that when the devastating earthquake of 1906 hit San Francisco, Italian homeowners on Telegraph Hill battled the fires that ensued with basement-stored barrels of red wine. Even so, wine consumption was largely confined to immigrant households until the postwar era, when the modern California wine industry began under the care of growers and vintners such as Robert Mondavi, Joe Rochioli, David Abreu, and many others.

That modern industry has a curious twist. Now, there are doubtless those who still think that French wine means Montrachet, while California wine means Thunderbird. Steven Spurrier, an English wine merchant transplanted to Paris, shared some of that prejudice, but he allowed himself to be pleasantly surprised when, in the early 1970s, visiting journalists and winemakers cajoled him to try some of the new breed of California varietals, which went far beyond what screw-top Paul Masson wines could offer. On a whim, Spurrier organized a blind tasting with a panel made up of France's best-known wine experts, among them the inspector general of the Appellation d'Origine Contrôlee Board and the editor of the *Revue du Vin de France*. A superb Chateau Montalena 1973 Chardonnay took top prize, grown in the rich soil of

Calistoga, California, at great remove from the prized terroir of Burgundy or Bordeaux.

French and American wines had been sharing tables for generations: It was American rootstock that saved the French wine industry in the nineteenth century, French grapes that elevated California wines above bathtub plonk. But it was a curious alchemy with a curious cast of characters, including a Chicago classicist who took up winemaking, a Croatian refugee who helped prove that Zinfandel originated in his homeland, and the children and grandchildren of Italian immigrants who insisted, against the suspicions of their Protestant neighbors, that drinking wine was a good thing, who made that industry whirl. The upshot of their labors, by the 1970s, was a magnificent California wine industry, despite an occasionally flooded market and the rise of such infra dig oddities as Two-Buck Chuck, and a scene much different from that of 1976, in which, as the wine journalist George M. Taber writes in his book *Judgment of Paris*, "the dynamic part of the world wine business today is not in Europe, but in the New World—Argentina, Australia, Chile, New Zealand, South Africa, and the United States."

Since the 1970s wine consumption in America has steadily risen; to name one measure, in 1993 American consumption stood at 1.74 gallons per capita, while in 2013 that figure had risen to 2.82 gallons. In 2014, to cite another measure, wines from California alone constituted a $25 billion industry, accounting for about 90 percent of all production in the United States.

Alcohol claims victims, of course. One, familiar to moviegoers around the world in his day, was Thomas Hezekiah Mix, one of Hollywood's hardest-working actors, who chalked up an astonishing career run of 336 feature films—all but nine of them silent. In 1940 when he was sixty and beginning to fade from the A list, he came to Tucson on a publicity tour. He received a crowd of fans at a downtown theater, then repaired to a bar and drank enough that he was reportedly asked to leave. Early the next morning, presumably worse for the wear, he headed to Phoenix in his Cord Roadster convertible along a narrow, rollercoaster highway that twists and turns its way across a landscape of steep-banked streambeds and low granite hills. When Mix, traveling at sixty miles an hour, swerved to avoid a road crew working on the banks of an arroyo, his car left the road and plowed into a clump of mesquite trees. He died instantly, it's said, his head crushed by a flying suitcase. His name was given to the wash almost immediately, and a memorial was later built near the site of the accident—an object lesson in sleeping it off, and certainly in not drinking and driving.

Tragedies are part and parcel of the whole alcoholic enterprise. But it is another of those rare human universals that our kind enjoys being delivered, from time to time, from our ordinary thoughts. Whether for purposes of religious transport, stress release, or simple enjoyment, alcohol has played a part in the human story from the very beginning, a story to which the Southwest has contributed more than its share.

12. The Future of Southwestern Food

Barrow, Alaska, is about as far from anywhere in North America as it's possible to get: hard by the Beaufort Sea; 720 miles from Anchorage; 3,500 miles from Washington, DC; 1,100 miles from the North Pole. Yet, until recently, it was possible to stumble across taiga and tundra and find, there in the heart of the town, a Mexican restaurant.

I say until recently, I say, because in 2013 Pepe's North of the Border, which billed itself as the northernmost Mexican restaurant in the world, burned to the ground. The owners plan to rebuild, they say, but for now the superlative belongs to some other establishment—perhaps in Nome, perhaps in Svalbard, perhaps somewhere that has yet to be known to anyone but a few hardy denizens of the Arctic.

Pepe's wasn't much, by all accounts; one review kindly remarked that it was "better than whale blubber." But then, when I was a teenager, then living in the Virginia suburbs of Washington, about the closest thing there was to Mexican food was a restaurant tucked away in a strip mall behind the state-run liquor store and a grocery, one whose idea of authenticity might have satisfied a cheese-loving Wisconsinite but would never have passed muster closer to the nation's southern border. It was better than whale blubber, too, but not by much.

Fast-forward forty years, and all that has changed. Today metropolitan Washington has dozens of Mexican restaurants—and supremely authentic ones at that, representing many of the regions of Mexico. In their commercial vanguard were establishments in the Southwestern style: Tex-Mex and Sonoran, that is, heavy on the beef that is produced in abundance in the border states of Chihuahua and Sonora, heavy on the flour tortillas that speak to the Sonoran breadbasket, vast wheat fields flanking the Gulf of California and the western flank of the Sierra Madre.

These restaurants were once largely confined to the gates of military posts, favored by soldiers, sailors, and aviators who had been stationed in Texas, New Mexico, Arizona, and Southern California and found themselves missing fire and spice. Over time, helped along by cartoonish Chihuahua dogs and mustachioed bandidos, they have become commonplace, so much so that you can scarcely find a town in America where it is not possible to get some approximation of Mexican food—taco Tuesdays in Providence, enchiladas in Paducah, even pretty decent tamales in Peoria and Pierre.

The ubiquity of Mexican food today, albeit mostly Mexican food of the Southwestern borderlands, speaks to both demographic and cultural shifts that were first made manifest in 1992—the five hundredth anniversary of the arrival of Christopher Columbus and crew in the Caribbean. In that year, perhaps fittingly, salsa outsold ketchup in the United States for the very first time. Fifteen years later, in 2007, reports the *Wall Street Journal*, it continued to outsell ketchup by a walloping $462.3 million to $298.9 million. (But, quibbled the venerable *Journal*, in terms of pounds moved, ketchup was the winner—as if sheer weight won anything other than pachydermatic contests.) This condiment gap, as a Kissingerian might call it, is due not only to the upswelling of immigration from Mexico and other Latino countries, though it certainly has something to do with that arrival, but also to a changing cuisine, with Mexican and other Hispanic foods assimilated just as fully as have been hot dogs, hamburgers, ketchup, pizza, and other once-exotic items in our larder. Call it the Southwesternization of the American palate.

In the 1930s, when good records of food sales were first kept, Mexican food was as exotic in most parts of the country as were actual Mexican people—who, outside the borderlands and Chicago, were rarely encountered. The first Anglo cookbooks to admit Mexican food did so gingerly and inauthentically: One from the early 1950s offered a recipe for tortillas that called for ordinary bread flour to be mixed with water, which would yield some-thing like a gluey pancake, an affront to anyone who knows what a real tor-tilla, cooked over wood fire atop a 55-gallon drum, is supposed to taste like. Not that anyone really knew, for even in Texas, soon to become a hotbed of borderland cuisine, chili powder was marketed as something that might be used to perk up a glass of tomato juice or liven up scrambled eggs, not the foundation on which to build a spicy meal.

In his memoir *Prime Green*, the late novelist Robert Stone recalls that in his Army boot-camp class, half the enlistees asked for a scoop of ice cream to accompany the strange thing called "pizza pie." The innocence was not confined to Italian food alone, for not until the 1970s was the taco—that great vanguard item of Mexican food—widely known north and east of Denver, allowing for a few immigrant pockets in places like Oklahoma City, Min-neapolis, and Detroit.

A decades-long influx of immigrants from Mexico and Central America, numbering many millions of arrivals widely distributed across the country, helped set the stage for a broadening of American taste, and if the main-stream attitude toward those people has often bordered on xenophobic hys-teria, their food has been much more readily accepted. At last count, there were more than fifty thousand Mexican restaurants across the country, including the outlets of numerous chains, and Mexican food represents the fastest-growing and largest segment of the ethnic foods market as reflected in what can be bought in an ordinary grocery store anywhere in the land.

Our xenophobia is not lessening, as we saw in the 2016 presidential cam-paign and its aftermath, but the American palate is now thoroughly South-westernized. We are just beginning to explore Mexican food, of course, for Mexican food goes far beyond the taco and the tamale, the toasted corn chip with the dollop of salsa. Consider, for example, birria, a kind of chili-infused stewed goat, beef, or pork usually served with lemon slices, radishes, and shredded cabbage with corn tortillas. A delicacy favored in Jalisco and other parts of central Mexico, birria connotes something like "slop"; served as a soup or in a liquidy taco with lime wedges, chile sauce, diced onions, and cilantro, it is held to be just the thing to cure or at least ameliorate a hangover. Birria was late in coming to many parts of the border; I first became aware of it when a former student of mine, a native of Guadalajara, opened a *birri-eria*, or birria restaurant, in Tucson in 1980. Now there are several such restaurants in Tucson. In Los Angeles where many Jaliscienses have migrated, there are dozens of birrierias, regularly contending for and winning critics' choice awards from food writers for the *Los Angeles Times* and the *LA Weekly*. The best of them are on the east side, while the best of them are on the west side in Chicago. But you can snag a bowl of birria in Boston and Seattle—and even my old hometown of Annandale, Virginia, which, though better known for its dozens of world-class Korean restaurants, doesn't lack for good food from the borderlands, either.

Our national taste has not yet opened much to the great variety of foods from farther south in Mexico, from head meat and spitted goat to chili-encrusted jicama and roast chicken covered in bitter chocolate. That may come in time, given the rapid spread of borderland food and the continuing growth of foodie culture: A decade from now, we may well be eating maguey-harvested ant larvae and corn smut, chayote and hojas de mora and huauzontle.

On a menu in Los Angeles recently, after all, I saw an entry for a taco with a filling of asparagus and cream cheese. If we're ready for that, it seems to me, then anything can happen and anything probably will.

Meanwhile, not long ago, I stopped in at a bakery in Fredericksburg, Texas, that fine old German freethinking town in the heart of the Hill Country, and ordered a kolache and coffee. The coffee was passable, for coffee remains a thing that this perfectible republic has yet to perfect universally. The kolache, though, was wonderful, a bit of Eastern Europe baked by a young woman from highland Mexico and served by another young woman from Cambodia, the shop owned by another immigrant from elsewhere in Southeast Asia. Men and women with numerous accents ordered pastries, some with a Texas twang, others with the telltale flatness of the mid-Atlantic, still others with the broad, swooping vowels of New York. And two women in their eighties spoke with the soft lilt of Texas German, an accent that is fast disappearing even as all these other voices fill the air.

The future of the food of the Southwest lies in this broad, ever-changing mix of newcomers and old communities, just as it always has. And though the forces of standardization and corporatization are hard at work in the region, just as they are everywhere on the planet, variations in local culture stubbornly persist: The chimichanga may have spread far and wide from its probable Sonora birthplace, but the bizcochito remains a New Mexican Hispano secret, the raja a specialty of the eastern borderland. Ask for a plate of enchiladas in Austin, and what arrives on your table will not be quite the plate of enchiladas that you will eat in Temecula, Tesuque, or Tacna.

Everything old is new again, and it comes to us on wheels. The first known food truck, at least of a kind we would recognize, dates to 1872, when an entrepreneur in Rhode Island, Walter Scott, sold lunches and coffee out of a wagon to passersby in downtown Providence. The "lunch wagon," as Scott called it, quickly spread, finally melding with the railroad dining car to become the immovable diner. In the early 1990s converted panel trucks and other vehicles began popping up on the south side of Tucson, motorized taquerias of Tucson and moveable feasts with fixed addresses. Modified vans, RVs, and utility trucks that sit on freshly poured concrete pads or alongside tile patios, these "taco wagons" offered delicacies not usually found in area restaurants, as my friend Hector Acuña and I discovered on a hot day in July 1995 when we decided, in the interest of journalistic comprehensiveness, to eat at as many of them as we could in a single day. One was a Chevy van bedecked with a cheesy mermaid-and-surfscape mural that turned out some fine, inexpensive seafood dishes: huge cocktails of scallops, shrimp, crab, and oysters; seafood tacos and burritos; and a first-rate ceviche tostada, with shellfish cooked in citrus juice and a light trace of peppers. Another, a step-van set under a broad-spreading paloverde tree, served up a mixed caldo studded with chunks of abalone, scallops, shrimp, and vegetables. A roadside santo shared the shade, commemorating the scene of a death a few years earlier, but it did not put us off our meal. Still another offered a stunning burrito of tripas de leche—cow innards, that is.

Our greatest discovery that day, and the hands-down winner in our quest, was a truck emblazoned with the name Papa Chino's, which served up the perfect syncretistic meal: the Sonoran hot dog. Now, archaeologists of food will argue long into the future about precisely who invented this concoction and when. All evidence points to an origin farther south than the Mexican state of Sonora, and the likelihood is that it stems from a food-cart snack served to construction workers in the Mexican capital as far back as the 1950s, when American manufacturers such as Oscar Meyer began to penetrate the lucrative Mexican market. Whatever the case, the Mexican or Sonoran hot dog makes use of the puffy brioche-style bun favored for what

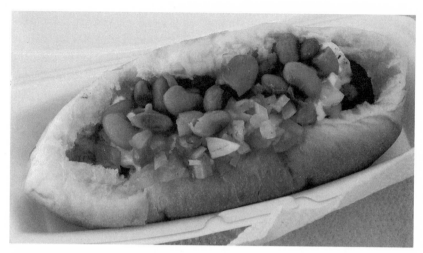

The Sonoran hot dog, a syncretic wonder.

are called lonches in Mexico, a step or two down on the hardness scale from the toothier German-inspired hot dog bun served north of the border. Blending another German innovation, the hot dog, with thick bacon courtesy of Mesopotamian pigs, Mediterranean onions, Central American beans, and Amazonian peppers and tomatoes, it makes for a guilty pleasure of the best kind, and a real treat for those unafraid of nitrates. Tucson remains the epicenter of the Sonoran hot dog in America, but it has spread, popularized by foodie television shows and converted into an object of food tourism.

Food trucks began popping up in Los Angeles at the same time, their spread stymied at times by overzealous health departments and a popular press inclined to tag them with the moniker "roach coaches." Most were operated by first-generation immigrants, a boon to foodies given the likelihood that the food they served was going to be authentic and unmediated by mainstream tastes. A few years later, though, as we saw in an earlier chapter, Roy Choi, born in South Korea in 1970, began to sell Korean-style tacos, making use of Korean barbecue and kimchi, in Los Angeles. It was largely through his efforts and growing renown, as commemorated by Jon Favreau's 2014 film *Chef,* that the food truck ascended from convenience to culturally desirable commodity.

Nearly every city in the Southwest has since embraced food truck culture, perhaps most notably Austin, Texas, which has whole mini-villages of the things tucked away among the tall trees of Lamar and South Congress Avenues. Los Angeles is also a world capital of mobile food, nourishing cultural blends that might seem unlikely elsewhere, as with Vietnamese American chef Hop Phan's truck Dos Chinos, with its blends such as curry chicken with sour cream and roast pork with salsa verde. Said one customer to *New York Times* writer Jennifer Medina of his three-year-old's food tastes, "My son is the only Mexican kid I know who says he wants rice and beans when he really means edamame and sushi rice. He eats food I never tasted growing up."

Tohono O'odham Hummus

Hummus is a longtime staple of Middle Eastern cuisines, but one that lends itself very nicely to ingredients from other traditions—in this instance, the Tohono O'odham of the Sonoran Desert. This dish figures on the seasonal menu of the Desert Rain Café in Sells, Arizona, the capital of the Tohono O'odham Nation.

2 cups cooked white tepary beans
¼ cup lemon juice
1 clove minced garlic
¼ teaspoon ground cumin
¼ cup extra virgin olive oil
2 teaspoons Sriracha, Tabasco, or other hot sauce (optional)
Reserve 1 cup of liquid from cooked beans.

Purée beans, lemon juice, and garlic in a blender or food processor. Stir in olive oil and cumin and purée until smooth. Add liquid from beans to thin to desired consistency. Add hot sauce to taste.

Meanwhile, our food networks expand apace. From the corn routes of Chaco Canyon to the intercontinental flights fueling the Tick-Tock Cafe is a long way, and those routes are becoming ever more extensive as North America begins to use South America and Oceania as its winter garden. Even as we begin to learn anew to eat locally, to grow our own food, to honor local traditions, we must increasingly recognize that there is something to what economists call economies of scale and the specialization of labor.

By way of experimentation, a foodie named Waldo Jaquith attempted to make a cheeseburger using only things he had produced himself, growing the vegetables, making the cheese, grinding the beef. As he wrote of the experiment,

> it's quite impractical—nearly impossible—to make a cheeseburger from scratch. Tomatoes are in season in the late summer. Lettuce is in season in spring and fall. Large mammals are slaughtered in early winter. The process of making such a burger would take nearly a year, and would inherently involve omitting some core cheeseburger ingredients. It would be wildly expensive—requiring a trio of cows—and demand many acres of land. There's just no sense in it.

Adds Jaquith, "A cheeseburger cannot exist outside of a highly developed, post-agrarian society." The same is true of a modern taco, or any other complex foodstuff. Getting one to our plates requires the interaction of farmers and vendors along a complicated chain of transactions. It requires transcontinental shipments, international treaties, customs clearances, email, texts, airports, roads, rail lines. It involves vast distances. If it is true that, as the German philosopher Ludwig Feuerbach put it, you are what you eat, then we are the products of centuries, continents, dozens of cultures: We are the world indeed.

That world, of course, is in trouble. Climate change, that great engine of human history, is upon the Southwest. With projected mean temperature increases of 5–10 degrees centigrade at the extreme, much of the region's water supply and consequent agriculture is threatened. It is tempting to look at a place such as Phoenix and imagine that, half a century from now, it will be as empty as Chaco Canyon, though presumably with better documentation on what caused its collapse.

The future is unwritten, to be sure, but it looks challenging, at the very least. To meet an exploding world population, to say nothing of a regional one, it is likely that our diets will have to change in a number of respects in the near future.

One of them would be nothing new to an Aztec, and it is the growing probability that we'll be eating insects in the near future—crickets, katydids, various sorts of beetles, ants. This prospect may be discomforting, of course, to many an American consumer, even if that insect protein comes to us disguised as part of the contents of a hamburger patty. (Never mind what our hamburgers *already* contain.) Given that the United Nations Food and Agriculture Organization has projected that the cost of meat will at least double between 2017 and 2025, a little insect filler may be a welcome cost-cutting device, and, in any event, scarcity and the vicissitudes of climate change may dictate that this measure will become commonplace. Insects are greatly more efficient at converting feed to meat than are cattle, and they contain much more protein by weight than cows, pigs, or birds—though "by weight" is an issue, since it would take a thousand crickets to yield the equivalent mass of a twelve-ounce steak.

Considering that we eat related sea creatures, it's not that far a jump. Says one analyst, "They will become popular when we get away from the word 'insects' and use something like 'mini-livestock.'"

We Southwesterners face increasing scarcities of water supplies, conditioning what we can grow and in what quantity, and perhaps occasioning the abandonment of crops long grown in the region but better suited to wetter climes, such as cotton and citrus—or cattle, for that matter. Some scarcities we can hardly begin to contemplate, such as a report by the American Chemical Society that the world's agricultural nations face impending shortages of phosphorus, a key ingredient in chemical fertilizer. "Resources of phosphate rock, mined to produce fertilizer, will be depleted within the next 30–100 years," the report warns, adding, "at present, no substitute exists for that natural source of phosphorous fertilizer." It does not help that major supplies of phosphate rock are located in the politically unstable desert nations of Morocco and Western Sahara, as well as the Taklimakan of Central Asia, places too often in the news for all the wrong reasons.

We face shortages of seafood, that great and seemingly inexhaustible resource that sustained so many tribes along the coasts of the Gulf of California, the Pacific Ocean, and the Gulf of Mexico. In the Gulf of California, the finger of the Pacific Ocean that makes the Sonoran Desert a maritime one, 90 percent of the populations of most large fish species have disappeared. Commercial fishers have harvested large predatory fish at the top of the oceanic food chain without concern for the effect this would have

218

on the ecosystem, putting the fish that we associate with Southwestern cuisine—snapper, sea bass, grouper, and such—onto our tables. Now the commercial fisheries have collapsed or are near doing so, not just for finfish but also for local shellfish such as shrimp. The ceviche we eat in Mexican restaurants these days is likelier to come from Alaska or Hawaii than from any nearby ocean, and, perhaps worse, is likely to be some extruded product of what gourmands once disdained as "trash fish." Richard C. Brusca, then of the Arizona-Sonora Desert Museum in Tucson, put it well of the local resource: "Fish from the Sea of Cortez, our Sonoran Desert ocean, remains an excellent choice for local healthy food. But we need to better manage our harvests and our consumption to prevent catastrophic collapse of marine ecosystems."

Grilled Fish Smoked with Bay Leaves

Published in 1898, Encarnación Pinedo's *El cocinero español* (*The Spanish Cook*) is a trove of Californio food lore and technique. We may live in a time of collapsing fisheries, but her recipe for grilled fish cries for a visit to the central coast, where bay laurels abound.

After cleaning the fish, wipe it dry and spread it with a mixture of salt, pepper, lemon juice, and olive oil.

Put it on the grill and place some bay leaves on the coals under it from time to time so the fish receives all the smoke.

Turn the fish frequently, basting it until golden.

Shortages loom, as they have throughout the history of this place: That the peoples of the ancient Southwest knew thousands of food plants was likely not a sign that they were gourmands, but that scarcity dictated diversification and an informed knowledge of what could be eaten without harm. Not for nothing is "agricultural rustling" an increasingly prevalent crime in the fields of California, with avocados, grapes, almonds, and even beehives stolen in record numbers. Not for nothing has the Chipotle Mexican restaurant chain even made contingency plans for the unthinkable: forgoing guacamole, given the shortage and expense of avocados, of which it reportedly uses thirty-five million pounds a year. (When I lived in Guadalajara, my porch was shaded by five avocado trees. Little did I realize then that it was paradise.) Not for nothing are almonds becoming ever more expensive as California growers battle other users for ever tighter supplies of agricultural water.

But, mini-livestock or no, rustled crops or no, scarcity or plenty, we waste an appalling amount of food. Simply reining that waste in can alleviate much of our impending burden.

One of the great contributions of contemporary Southwestern archaeology was born when I was an undergraduate: the University of Arizona's Garbage Project—or Projet du Garbage, as we affectionately called it. The brainchild of Mesoamerican archaeologist William Rathje, the Garbage Project was an innovative application of archaeology to contemporary society—that old ethnographic analogy brought to life. If modern household waste could be examined, what might it tell us about the nutritional habits, social organization, wealth, political standing, even religious beliefs of those who threw it away? So it was that for day after fetid day, we undergraduate anthropology students stood in Tucson's main garbage dump and counted cheese wrappers, bones, rotting cucumbers, and beer cans, comparing these hard data to what the people who discarded them said about their lives—stories that had them eating more healthfully and certainly drinking less than their artifacts betold.

What we can say from the data is that the average American family of four effectively is withdrawing $3,000 from the bank and throwing it into the nearest garbage can each year. That's no exaggeration: as of 2015, the average family of four spends a bit more than $10,000 a year on food, give or take. Astonishingly, shockingly, that same family throws out somewhere between one-fourth and one-half of the food it purchases—a figure that, strangely, has steadily risen since statistics were first kept in the 1970s, in part because of the Garbage Project's data, and increasing even during our recent times of economic turmoil. Multiply 310 million Americans by the three dollars that each throws away in spoiled or uneaten food each day, and you have enough to fund the space program, give every child on the planet a college education, replace nearly every bridge and every mile of road in the United States— enough money to make a big difference in the world, in other words.

Consider the problem in another way. It takes more than six tons of water to produce a pound of beef. Every uneaten bite represents squandered water. Every uneaten bite of food of whatever kind represents wasted agricultural land. It also represents a huge amount of wasted energy: even the low end of the estimated annual food loss represents more gas and oil than is produced in the United States in the same period of time.

Think of it still another way. Each of us Americans, on average, throws away about half a pound of food a day, or 197 pounds of food a year. Taken nationwide, that's 160 billion pounds of food a year—enough to fill a professional football stadium twice over.

Why do we waste so much food? For one thing, we simply buy too much of it, partly because most of us travel by car to buy groceries, since the average American lives a little more than two miles from the nearest food store. That trip must seem a chore, for we try to do it only every week or so, which makes a recipe for overbuying. Americans at large have come to desire quantity over quality, it seems; even with the widespread trimming of portion sizes and package weights in restaurants and stores in response to the Great Recession, our food is simply too big. Any restaurant dishwasher can tell you how much food gets tossed away from a dinner plate—but any restaurateur can also tell you that efforts to bring portion control to food service usually result in squawking.

The two categories in which most food waste occurs are dairy products and vegetables. Curiously, so it has always been: in the days when refrigeration was iffy or not available at all, much milk and much vegetable food went to livestock when deemed no longer safe or appetizing for human consumption.

Can we mend our wasteful ways? You have not lived until you have pondered this question in the full heat of a desert day amid torn-open plastic bags full of decomposing hamburger and green beans, with a full diaper or two thrown in for good measure. The answer is: Certainly. We don't waste food because we're bad people. We waste food because we're unaware that we're doing so, never having been taught to think about it, or because we imagine ourselves to live in unfettered abundance. That will probably be fettered soon enough, in part by necessity, but, more positively, in part because more and more of us are turning to local growing, buying closer to home and in smaller quantity, raising our own vegetables. We can all stand to lose a little weight, after all—and a recent Canadian study found that people who live within two-thirds of a mile from a grocery store weigh 11 percent less than those who live farther away, suggesting that there's room for a healthful food vendor on every corner. The supersized meals of our time have yielded supersized

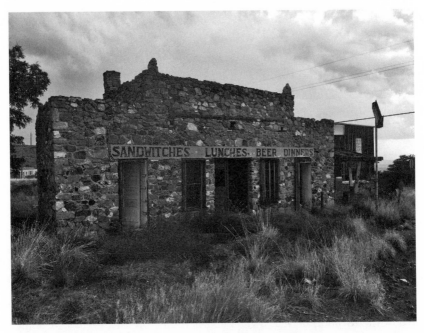

The old cycle of boom and bust defines the Southwest, as this unfortunate former diner in the Organ Mountains of New Mexico suggests.

humans; it's worth noting that the average adult American man in 1850, the time of the first Anglo arrivals in the Southwest, weighed about 146 pounds, a full 50 pounds less than the average American male weighed in 2015.

Granted, we stand several inches taller and live thirty years longer. Times change, people change, and our world changes. One little measure is, I think, a happy one with which to close this unhappy meditation on scarcity and waste, and that is this: It wasn't that long ago that chickens were animals non grata in the backyards of Los Angeles, Tucson, Las Cruces, and San Antonio. Community and private gardens are now everywhere. Now we can awaken to the sound of crowing at every dawn and gather food just outside our doors, a return to the past in the most positive of ways, a sign of changing times and of greater connection to the food we eat for our survival and our pleasure.

To complain about food is to risk seeming a little ungallant, for we have come a very far way even as we have circled back. Forty years ago, when I first began to crisscross the country in quest of good things to eat, it was tough to find a decent cup of coffee or an edible loaf of bread in most of America. Now it is possible to find a fine cup of espresso in small towns such as Ellensburg, Washington; Luray, Virginia; and Alamogordo, New Mexico. I know, because I have drunk them there. Ordinary supermarkets carry good French bread and Viennese pastries. I know, because I have eaten altogether too many of them, as my increasingly Hitchcockian look will attest. Ethnic groceries abound, and chains such as Whole Foods and Trader Joe's are introducing harried urbanites to the notion that eating from a microwave, while barbarous to card-carrying foodies, can make for some pleasant evenings.

If it's still not always easy to get a leafy salad out on the Great Plains, where gelatin counts as a substitute, acceptable Chinese, Mexican, and Italian eateries dot the landscape, which, by the standards of three decades past, is nothing short of miraculous. Never mind, as Charles Baker-Clark huffs in *Profiles from the Kitchen*, that the waiter at the local Italian chain outlet "probably does not know very much beyond what he may have been spoon-fed by the corporation that owns the restaurant." At least we can get something other than meat loaf and calf fries, and that is victory enough.

That American foodways have changed so markedly in such a relatively short time is the work of brilliant chefs and food activists such as James Beard, Julia Child, Rick Bayless, and John T. Edge, to name just a few. They are our heroes, the men and women who stood up and said, resoundingly, no to the fast, tasteless food that still stuffs the national face, the ones who make a mockery of mall-rat travesties that serve up pseudo-ethnic food that no one in any self-respecting nation would actually eat. Consider one such monstrosity, as Baker-Clark growls: "refried beans laced with lard and topped with processed melted cheese and sour cream." Now, I have actually seen just such a thing being consumed in a fine and authentic restaurant in Guadalajara, Mexico, but I did not stop to question whether the diner was an improvisationally minded, calorie-starved gringo or someone defying expectation by doing what the natives are not supposed to do. No matter: In foodist law, lard-laced refrieds are fine, lard-laced refrieds covered with processed cheese are a crime.

We learn as much by following the path of Carlo Petrini, the founder of the much-needed Slow Food Movement, and learning to take the time to investigate what it is we are putting into our mouths and stomachs. We take the point by hanging out with Angus Campbell, who reassures his fellow cooks that it's all right to take your eyes off an onion in the frying pan and "simply leave the food alone for a period of time." We broaden our minds (and perhaps our midriffs) by taking Susan Spicer's example and learning by doing—in this case, by spending hours upon untold hours in the kitchen actually cooking, not simply gaping at celebrity-cook television shows.

And let us not forget the noble efforts of the late, great American novelist and gourmand Jim Harrison, with whom I shared many fine sessions at table and who reminds us in his marvelous book *The Raw and the Cooked* that there are meals worth hopping in a beat-up car and driving thousands of miles cross-country to eat. To confine it just to our region, a grain-fed steak in Dallas, sushi in Los Angeles, crabs in Morro Bay, red chile in Phoenix and green in Albuquerque, and maybe a bratwurst or two in New Braunfels.

These are our heroes, as I say. We have every reason to be thankful to them, and to the wild-eyed food radicals behind such at-root conservative groups as Native Seeds and the New Mexico FoodShed Alliance, the food-truck chefs of Los Angeles and Austin, the Bioneers and, way back when, the Diggers. It is the makers of food, the growers and truckers and cooks, who ultimately make it possible for us to eat decently just about anywhere—not that we always do. The success of those makers of food has been astonishing. It has been food, more than anything else, that has revitalized the down-towns of nearly every Southwestern city, food that has quickened local and regional economies. Sometimes success has been a bit too much, though surely not too soon: Witness the recent "brisket boom" in Austin, in which those toothy pectoral muscles were selling for double what they had been just a few years earlier and knowing diners were camping out all night at places like Franklin Barbecue lest supplies run out before they could claim a bite. And not just Austin; as business writer Ana Campoy reports in the *Wall Street Journal*, "Foodies are stampeding to restaurants in New York, Chicago and San Francisco, waiting in long lines to secure a few slices from a true practitioner of the smoking arts. Connoisseurs are embarking on barbecue-joint pilgrimages, ingesting pounds of meat a day and waxing eloquent about its perfectly rendered fat and crusty exterior." Even in the face of localism, then, the very Southwesternization of the American palate may be producing shortages all on its own.

The future cuisine of the Southwest will likely have us making do with a

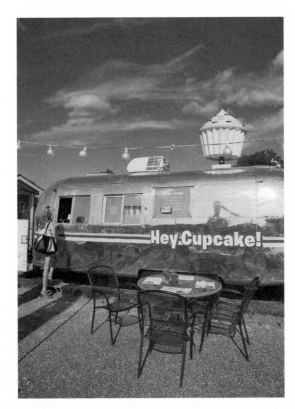

The food trucks of Austin, Texas, beckon.

little less, which may in turn yield unexpected plenty. If we are lucky and persistent, it will turn on continuing to revive lost food traditions—corn smut and insects, perhaps, but also amaranth and tepary beans, mesquite flour and verdolagas, and a thousand other things. We will almost certainly be eating corn; researchers at the Autonomous National University of Mexico have optimistically announced that transgenic breeds of corn can survive a changing climate and even thrive. With its reported fifty-nine landraces and more than two hundred varieties of corn, Mexico is better prepared than the comparatively genetically impoverished United States to contend with a drier, hotter future. As always, the Southwest has much to learn from its neighbor.

We will be seeing new syncretisms and new experiments. Some of the best sushi I have ever had has been made by Japanese Mexican chefs in places like Mexicali and Tijuana, with vinegared rice and deftly sliced fish set off with just a hint of chile. I can only begin to imagine what awaits as chefs in Los Angeles wed the traditions of, say, Iran to Mesoamerica, as Hmong flavors enter tamales and pizza finds toppings even more imaginative than the Mexican favorite of ham and pineapple.

If we are attentive to our history, we may deepen our understanding of traditional Native foods that were eaten before the arrival of Europeans: corn, beans, chiles, bison, rabbit, and so much more. Native American chefs are doing just that, developing what has been called a precolonization menu that does without white flour, processed sugar, dairy products, and meats such as beef, chicken, and pork. As the British newspaper *The Guardian* notes, with no small sense of wonder, Nambé Pueblo, near Santa Fe, has been feeding its elderly by means of a community farm producing just such foods, while a young Navajo chef named Freddie Bitsoie has been filming early episodes of a cooking show, *Rezervations Not Required*, that will explain, finally, how the food of Native America is as various as the food of the European culture surrounding it. In an odd way, after all, Native American cuisine is the last of the world's great cuisines to enjoy a true revival, to become a nouvelle cuisine that is very ancient, a circle that we have yet to close.

For the time being, we make do, we do, and we do well in varying degrees. It may be impossible to make a cheeseburger from scratch in one's home, but it is a pleasure to make one's way to New Mexico, find an eatery on the state's newly inaugurated Green Chile Cheeseburger Trail, and dig in. If Southwestern civilization truly does collapse, then I can imagine many worse places to see out the apocalypse than Sparky's in Hatch, the Largo Cafe in Quemado, or the Owl Bar in San Antonio—with enough gas in the tank, one hopes, to get to Pie Town and a last slice of apple-green chile pie.

There's a lot of eating to be done between now and then, lots of tortillas, tiswin, T-bones—and tacos and tamales and timbales and tinga and tandoor and tempura. I wish you the heartiest and healthiest of appetites.

Acknowledgments

This book began to take shape, fittingly, over tacos at a crowded, noisy restaurant on San Antonio's Riverwalk in the early winter of 2010. A few bites in, a few napkins scribbled on, and the basic shape of the book formed. It took several years for it to fall together, years occupied by other books, hundreds of periodical pieces, travels up and down and across the continent, and many other projects.

But how long have I been writing this book? All my life. I cannot remember a time before cooking, before reading, almost before writing, and in all those things I was taught by a thousand masters. Thousands of books, thousands of meals, thousands of people contributed to the experiences called forth in writing this book. To name any of those people is to risk forgetting to name others, so I will say here only that I thank all those who helped, the honor and the pleasure is all mine. Everyone who has shared a stovetop, a table, a campstool, a bumpy road, a reference, a recipe—you know who you are. Nods at those who did *not* help—you know who you are, too. I learned something from everyone, and so my thanks are sincere to all concerned.

Please visit the website for this book, www.ancientsouthwest.com. There, I'll post news related to it, along with oddments that I think might be worth your attention. Please feel free to drop a note there. Let me know what I missed, remembering the nonfiction writer's mantra: "I'll correct it in the next edition."

Many thanks for reading this book. *¡Buen provecho!*

References

General

Brothwell, Dan, and Patricia Brothwell. *Food in Antiquity*. Baltimore: Johns Hopkins University Press, 1998.

Carroll, Abigail. *Three Squares: The Invention of the American Meal*. New York: Basic Books, 2013.

Fernández-Armesto, Felipe. *Near a Thousand Tables: A History of Food*. New York: Free Press, 2002.

Graff, Sarah R., and Enrique Rodríguez-Alegría. *The Menial Art of Cooking: Archaeological Studies of Cooking and Food Preparation*. Boulder: University Press of Colorado, 2012.

Hicks, Jack, James D. Houston, Maxine Hong Kingston, and Al Young, eds. *The Literature of California: Writings from the Golden State*. Berkeley: University of California Press, 2000.

Chapter 1

Peacock, Doug. *In the Shadow of the Sabertooth*. Chico, CA: AK Press, 2013.

Wrangham, Richard. *Catching Fire: How Cooking Made Us Human*. New York: Basic Books, 2010.

Chapter 2

Andrews, Jean. *The Pepper Trail: History and Recipes from Around the World*. College Station: Texas A&M University Press, 2001.

Barrows, David Prescott. *Ethno-botany of the Coahuilla Indians*. Banning, CA: Malki Museum, 1967.

Brown, Cecil H., Charles R. Clement, Patience Epps, Eike Luedeling, and Søren Wichmann. "The Paleobiolinguistics of Domesticated Chili Pepper (Capsicum spp.)." *Ethnobiology Letters* 4 (2013): 1–11.

Burns, Barney T. "A Short History of Panic Grass." *Seedhead News* (Spring 2011): 6–7.

Ebeling, Walter. *Handbook of Indian Foods and Fibers in Arid America*. Berkeley: University of California Press, 1986.

Hill, Jane H. "Proto-Uto-Aztecan as a Mesoamerican Language." *Ancient Mesoamerica* 23 (2012): 57–68.

Kaplan, Lawrence. "The Cultivated Beans of the Prehistoric Southwest." *Annals of the Missouri Botanical Garden* 43, no. 2 (May 1956): 189–251.

Krieger, Alex D. *We Came Naked and Barefoot: The Journey of Cabeza de Vaca Across North America*. Austin: University of Texas Press, 2003.

MacLachlan, Colin M. *Imperialism and the Origins of Mexican Culture*. Cambridge, MA: Harvard University Press, 2015.

Rancho Santa Ana Botanic Garden. *Native Partners: Plants & Peoples of California*. Claremont, CA: RSABG, 2010.

Staller, J. E., R. H. Tykot, and B. F. Benz, eds. *Histories of Maize: Multidisciplinary Approaches to the Prehistory, Biogeography, Domestication, and Evolution of Maize*. Amsterdam: Elsevier, 2006.

Staller, John L. *Maize Cobs and Cultures: History of Zea mays L.* Berlin: Springer Verlag, 2010.

Vaillant, G. C. *Aztecs of Mexico*. London: Penguin, 1950.

Wheat, Margaret. *Survival Arts of the Primitive Paiutes*. Reno: University of Nevada Press, 1967.

Chapter 3

Arciniegas, Germán. *Caribbean: Sea of the New World*. New York: Knopf, 1946.

Bernstein, William J. *A Splendid Exchange: How Trade Shaped the World*. New York: Grove Press, 2008.

Columbus, Christopher. *The Four Voyages*. Translated by J. M. Cohen. London: Penguin, 1969.

Cortés, Hernán. *Conquest: Dispatches of Cortés from the New World*. Edited by Irwin R. Blacker and Harry M. Rosen. New York: Grosset, 1962.

Crosby, Alfred W. *Ecological Imperialism: The Biological Expansion of Europe, 900–1900*. Cambridge: Cambridge University Press, 1986.

Davies, R. Trevor. *The Golden Century of Spain, 1501–1621*. New York: Harper & Row, 1937.

de Sahagún, Bernardino. *Florentine Codex: General History of the Things of New Spain*. Salt Lake City: University of Utah Press, 2012.

Dunmire, William M. *Gardens of New Spain: How Mediterranean Plants and Foods Changed America*. Austin: University of Texas Press, 2004.

Dutton, Davis, ed. *Missions of California*. New York: Ballantine, 1972.

Kroeber, A. L. *Handbook of the Indians of California*. Washington, DC: US Bureau of Ethnology, 1919.

Laudan, Rachel. *Cuisine & Empire: Cooking in World History*. Berkeley: University of California Press, 2013.

Riley, Carroll L. *The Kachina and the Cross: Indians and Spaniards in the Early Southwest*. Salt Lake City: University of Utah Press, 1999.

Sheridan, Thomas E. "The Limits of Power: The Political Ecology of the Spanish Empire in the Greater Southwest." *Antiquity* 66 (1992): 133–71.

Weber, David J. *The Spanish Frontier in North America*. New Haven, CT: Yale University Press, 1992.

Wolf, Eric R. *Europe and the People Without History*. Berkeley: University of California Press, 1982.

Yetman, David. "Pedro de Perea and the Colonization of Sonora." *Journal of the Southwest* 53, no. 1 (Spring 2011): 33–87.

Chapter 4

Cisneros, Sandra. *Caramelo*. New York: Knopf, 2002.

Fergusson, Erna. *Mexican Cookbook*. Albuquerque: University of New Mexico Press, 1945.

Johnson, Ronald. *Southwestern Cooking New & Old*. Albuquerque: University of New Mexico Press, 1985.

Officer, James O. *Hispanic Arizona, 1536–1856*. Tucson: University of Arizona Press, 1987.

Pinedo, Encarnación. *Encarnación's Kitchen: Mexican Recipes from Nineteenth-Century California*. Berkeley: University of California Press, 2003.

Tolbert, Frank X. *A Bowl of Red*. College Station: Texas A&M University Press, 1953.

Valle, Victor M., and Mary Lau Valle. *Recipe of Memory: Five Generations of Mexican Cuisine*. New York: New Press, 1995.

Véa, Alfredo, Jr. *La Maravilla*. New York: Plume, 1993.

Chapter 5

Danbom, David D. *Born in the Country: A History of Rural America*. Baltimore: Johns Hopkins University Press, 1995.

Horsman, Reginald. *Feast or Famine: Food and Drink in American Westward Expansion.* Columbia: University of Missouri Press, 2008.

Lamar, Howard R. *The Far Southwest, 1846–1912: A Territorial History.* Albuquerque: University of New Mexico Press, 2000.

Nugent, Walter. *Into the West.* New York: Knopf, 1999.

Trigger, Bruce G., and Wilcomb Washburn, eds. *The Cambridge History of the Native Peoples of the Americas.* Cambridge: Cambridge University Press, 1996.

Williams, Jacqueline. *Wagon Wheel Kitchens: Food on the Oregon Trail.* Lawrence: University Press of Kansas, 1993.

Chapter 6

Clemings, Russell. *Mirage: The False Promise of Desert Agriculture.* Oakland, CA: Sierra Club Books, 1996.

Dawson, Carol, and Carol Johnston. *House of Plenty: The Rise, Fall, and Revival of Luby's Cafeterias.* Austin: University of Texas Press, 2006.

Fried, Stephen. *Appetite for America: Fred Harvey and the Business of Civilizing the Wild West —One Meal at a Time.* New York: Bantam Books, 2010.

Hagenstein, Edwin C., Sara M. Gregg, and Brian Donohue, eds. *American Georgics: Writings on Farming, Culture, and the Land.* New Haven, CT: Yale University Press, 2011.

Hanson, Victor Davis. *Fields Without Dreams: Defending the Agrarian Idea.* New York: Free Press, 1996.

Ingram, B. Lynn, and Frances Malamud-Roam. *The West Without Water: What Past Floods, Droughts, and Other Climatic Clues Tell Us about Tomorrow.* Berkeley: University of California Press, 2013.

Masumoto, David Mas. *Epitaph for a Peach.* New York: HarperCollins, 1995.

Morris, Roy, Jr. *Lighting Out for the Territory: How Samuel Clemens Headed West and Became Mark Twain.* New York: Simon & Schuster, 2010.

Palmer, Joel. *Journal of Travels Over the Rocky Mountains.* Glendale, CA: Arthur H. Clark, 1906.

Starr, Kevin. *Golden Dreams: California and the Age of Abundance, 1950–1963.* New York: Oxford University Press, 2009.

Starrs, Paul F. *Let the Cowboy Ride: Cattle Ranching in the American West.* Baltimore: Johns Hopkins University Press, 1998.

White, Richard. *Railroaded: The Transcontinentals and the Making of Modern America.* New York: Norton, 2011.

Chapter 7

Bower, Anne L., ed. *African American Foodways: Explorations of History & Culture.* Champaign: University of Illinois Press, 2007.

Harris, Jessica B. *High on the Hog: A Culinary Journey from Africa to America.* New York: Bloomsbury Books, 2011.

Miller, Adrian. *Soul Food.* Chapel Hill: University of North Carolina Press, 2013.

Moss, Robert F. *Barbecue: The History of an American Institution.* Tuscaloosa: University of Alabama Press, 2010.

Nash, Gerald D. *The American West Transformed: The Impact of the Second World War.* Bloomington: Indiana University Press, 1985.

Tipton-Martin, Toni. *The Jemima Code: Two Centuries of African American Cookbooks.* Austin: University of Texas Press, 2015.

Chapter 8

Deutsch, Jonathan, and Rachel Saks. *Jewish American Food Culture.* Lincoln: University of Nebraska Press, 2009.

Diner, Hasia R. *Hungering for America: Italian, Irish & Jewish Foodways in the Age of Migration.* Cambridge, MA: Harvard University Press, 2001.

Dutkova-Cope, Lida. "Texas Czech Ethnic Identity: So How Czech Are You, Really?" *Slavic and East European Journal* 47, no 4. (Winter 2003): 648–76.

Kahn, Ava F., ed. *Jewish Life in the American West.* Los Angeles: Autry Museum of Western Heritage, 2002.

Ornish, Natalie. *Pioneer Jewish Texans.* College Station: Texas A&M University Press, 2011.

Rios, Alberto. *Capirotada.* Albuquerque: University of New Mexico Press, 1999.

Rochlin, Harriet, and Fred Rochlin. *Pioneer Jews: A New Life in the Far West.* New York: Houghton Mifflin, 1984.

Tobias, Henry J. *A History of the Jews in New Mexico.* Albuquerque: University of New Mexico Press, 1990.

Chapter 9

Coe, Andrew. *Chop Suey: A Cultural History of Chinese Food in the United States.* New York: Oxford University Press, 2009.

Rath, Eric C., and Stephanie Assmann, eds. *Japanese Foodways Past and Present.* Champaign: University of Illinois Press, 2010.

Chapter 10

Collingham, Lizzie. *The Taste of War: World War II and the Battle for Food.* New York: Penguin Press, 2012.

Doolin, Kaleta. *Fritos Pie.* College Station: Texas A&M University Press, 2011.

Hines, Duncan. *The Dessert Book.* Macon, GA: Mercer University Press, 2002.

Horowitz, Roger. *Putting Meat on the American Table: Taste, Technology, Transformation.* Baltimore: Johns Hopkins University Press, 2006.

Pilcher, Jeffrey M. "Who Chased out the 'Chili Queens'? Gender, Race, and Urban Reform in San Antonio, Texas, 1880–1943." *Food & Foodways* 16 (2008): 173–200.

Root, Waverley. *The Paris Edition.* San Francisco: North Point Press, 1987.

Chapter 11

Fish, Suzanne K., Paul R. Fish, Charles Miksicek, and John Madsen. "Prehistoric Agave Cultivation in Southern Arizona." *Desert Plants* 7, no. 2 (1985): 107–112.

Gentry, Howard Scott. *Agaves of Continental North America*. Tucson: University of Arizona Press, 1982.

Hodgson, Wendy C., and Andrew M. Salywon. "Two New Agave Species (Agavaceae) from Central Arizona and Their Putative Pre-Columbian Domesticated Origins." *Brittonia* 65 (2013): 5–15.

Holmes, Kenneth L., ed. *Covered Wagon Women: Diaries and Letters from the Western Trail*. Glendale, CA: Arthur H. Clarke, 1983.

Martineau, Chantal. *How the Gringos Stole Tequila*. Chicago: Chicago Review, 2015.

Sipos, Ed. *Brewing Arizona: A Century of Beer in the Grand Canyon State*. Tucson: University of Arizona Press, 2013.

Taber, George M. *Judgment of Paris: California vs. France and the Historic 1976 Paris Tasting That Revolutionized Wine*. New York: Scribner, 2005.

Chapter 12

Choi, Roy. *L.A. Son: My Life, My City, My Food*. New York: Ecco, 2013.

Goodyear, Dana. "The Missionary," *The New Yorker*, January 30, 2012.

Index

7-Eleven, 180

A&W, 184
acorn, 33, 55
Acuña, Rodolfo, 80
African Americans in Southwest, 8, 31,
    127–39, 155, 158
agarita, 33
agave, 23, 28, 39, 46, 68, 191–97, 199
Akimel O'odham, vii, 17, 19, 26, 29, 36,
    45, 124–25
albondigas, 120
Albuquerque, New Mexico, 54, 64, 67,
    124, 168, 178, 186, 223
Alibates Flint Quarries, Texas, 15
almond, 47, 59, 125–26, 218, 219
amaranth, 23–25, 35, 38, 76, 142, 224
America Is in the Heart (memoir by
    Carlos Bulosan), 166
Anaheim, California, 151, 162
Ancestral Pueblo, 10, 23, 29, 40, 126
antelope. *See* pronghorn
Apache people, 7, 17, 33, 57, 93, 94, 115,
    129, 193, 200
apple, 49, 59, 60, 61, 63, 64, 72, 110, 116,
    122, 225

apple pie, New Mexico, 60, 225
Arizona, x, xi, 8, 14, 17, 19, 24, 29, 35, 36,
    45, 55, 59, 70, 74, 75, 76, 77, 79, 84,
    92–93, 94, 98, 101, 102, 107, 113, 114,
    115, 116, 117, 120, 122, 123, 124, 134,
    141, 142, 144, 146, 149, 150, 158, 159,
    161, 162, 168, 180, 184, 185, 186, 193,
    195, 196, 201, 203, 204, 210, 215, 218
Arkansas, 80, 138
Austin, Texas, 11, 71, 124, 133, 172, 180,
    204, 213, 215, 223, 224
avocado, ix, 44, 79, 122, 124, 143, 167,
    218–19
Aztecs, 21, 24, 25–29, 34, 40, 44, 45, 47,
    129, 171, 216

Baja California, Mexico, 3, 39, 69, 122,
    161
barbecue, 134–37, 144, 171, 172, 185, 214,
    223
basil, 49, 66, 76, 109
Bat Cave, New Mexico, 27, 39
Bayless, Rick, 148, 196, 199, 222
beans, ix, xii, 35, 36, 38, 39, 45, 46, 47, 55,
    57, 64, 66, 69, 70, 71, 72, 73, 74, 75,
    76, 77, 79, 98, 99, 102, 119, 131, 155,

Index

beans (*continued*)
163, 182, 187, 214, 215, 220, 222, 224, 225; refried, 45, 46, 47, 69, 75, 76, 187, 222
bear, 8, 11, 12, 13, 81, 132, 151
beer, 80, 133, 151, 180, 183, 200, 202–4, 219
Bering land bridge, 1
Beringia, 3, 11
Billy the Kid (William Bonney), 94–96
birria, 211–12
bison, 8, 11, 14, 15, 22, 29, 30, 31, 56, 98, 99, 225
Blackwater Draw, New Mexico, 8, 10, 14
Boone, Daniel, 81–83, 84, 88, 187
Bowden, Charles, 169–70
Boy Scouts, 85–86
Brusca, Richard, 39, 218
Burbank, Luther, 108–12
Burke, Edmund, 84, 89

Cabeza de Vaca, Álvar Núñez, 31–32, 39, 54, 129, 145
caesar salad, 175–76, 190
calabacitas, 74
California roll, 167
California, ix, x, xi, 13, 14, 15, 23, 33, 39, 48, 49, 57, 60, 71, 72, 73, 79, 80, 85, 88, 90, 92, 93, 98, 106, 109, 110, 112, 113, 114, 115, 116, 117, 118, 121, 122, 123, 124, 126, 127, 128, 130, 138, 143, 144, 149, 151, 152, 158, 158, 159, 160, 162, 163, 165, 166, 168, 172, 173, 175, 179, 180, 184, 185, 186, 189, 191, 196, 199, 201, 202, 203, 205, 206, 210, 219
camel, 8, 11, 13, 14, 149, 150
Capitorada (memoir by Alberto Ríos), 155–56
Caramelo (novel by Sandra Cisneros), xi–xii
Cardini, Cesare, 175–76
Carpenter, John, 21
Casa Grande, Arizona, 35, 168

Castro, Rosaura, 75–76
cattle, ix, 6, 10, 48, 49–50, 54, 56–57, 68, 72, 73, 92–93, 94, 96–97, 106, 121, 127, 144–45, 146, 149, 216, 217
Chaco Canyon, New Mexico, 20, 29–30, 39–40, 215, 216
Chandler, Raymond, 106
cheese, ix, 50–51, 64, 71, 74, 77, 79, 100, 120, 121, 153, 156, 175, 176, 178, 180, 182, 212
cheeseburger, 216, 225
cherry, 38, 59, 110
chia, 25, 46
chicken, vii, 9, 24, 47, 48, 56, 66, 70, 75, 79, 80, 99, 100, 101, 121, 130, 133, 134, 136, 138, 143, 146, 151, 159, 169, 185, 187, 190, 212, 215, 221, 225
chicken fried steak, 151–52
Chihuahua, Mexico, 7, 51, 52, 69, 153, 194, 210
Chihuahua cheese, 51
Chihuahuan Desert, 37, 191
chile, xii, 36, 37, 38, 39, 40, 44, 59, 60, 66, 67–71, 75, 77, 78, 79, 96, 132, 144, 147, 155, 162, 164, 182, 186, 187, 194, 198, 211, 223, 225
chile colorado, 68, 70, 96, 102
chili con carne, 70, 151, 187
chimichanga, 75, 77, 152, 212
Chinese in Southwest, 121, 155, 157–62, 165, 166, 169, 170, 172, 222
chocolate, 40, 41, 43, 47, 54, 56, 66, 79, 212
Choi, Roy, 171, 214
climate, xi, 12, 48, 49, 51–54, 64, 73, 76, 105, 106, 108, 117, 122, 169, 202
climate change, viii, 3, 4–6, 7–8, 12–14, 48, 51–54, 108, 216–17, 224
Clovis culture, 8, 10–15, 17, 21
Cochiti Pueblo, 16
coffee, 49, 58, 90, 96, 98, 102, 118, 144, 146, 154, 158, 213, 222
Colorado, x, xi, 13, 86, 98

Colorado River, xi, 32, 117, 123, 141, 150, 151, 186

Columbian exchange, 43, 60, 63, 66, 132

Columbus, Christopher, 43–44, 47, 48, 49, 53, 54, 63, 76, 116, 134, 142, 143, 210

corn, viii, xi, 6, 8, 20, 21, 24, 25–28, 30, 32, 33, 34–36, 38, 39, 40, 43, 46, 47, 52, 54, 55, 56, 57, 58, 61, 63, 64, 66, 68, 71, 72, 73, 74, 79, 80, 93, 96, 98, 99, 101, 110, 119, 121, 131, 132–33, 137, 138, 144, 147, 149, 154, 179, 181, 182, 183, 198, 199, 200, 204, 211, 212, 215, 220, 224, 225

corn dodgers, 96

Coronado, Francisco de, 54, 129

Cortés, Hernán, 21, 41, 44–47, 48, 53, 54, 58, 129, 132

cow. See cattle

coyote, 19–21, 22, 26, 50, 191

crab, 39, 165, 167, 213, 223

Crespi, Juan, 58, 60, 105

Crisco, 145

Czechs in Southwest, 136, 152–53

Danes in Southwest, 152

date, 12, 61, 122

Dateland, Arizona, 122

Death Comes for the Archbishop (novel by Willa Cather), 102

deer, 8, 11, 20, 22, 31, 38, 39, 85, 132, 134

delicatessen, 146–47

Disney, Walt, 83, 151, 185

dog, 21, 22, 201

domestication, xiii, ix, 23, 26, 32, 35, 36, 50, 135

Ehrenberg, Herman, 150–51

El Paso, Texas, 2, 17, 54, 57, 64, 115, 121, 124, 129, 161, 186, 205

enchilada, 121, 168, 187, 213

Estevánico, 31, 128–29

fajitas, 71

fig, 59, 61, 116

Filipinos in Southwest, 155, 157, 166, 172, 173

fish, 22, 38, 39, 43, 44, 69, 73–74, 77, 120, 132–33, 134, 163, 165, 167, 190, 217–18

Folsom culture, 8

food trucks, 172–73, 214–15

French in Southwest, 57, 102, 154, 205, 206

frijoles. See beans

Frito-Lay, 182

Frito pie, 182

Gadsden Purchase, 151

Gentry, Howard Scott, 193

Germans in Southwest, 150–52

Gila River, 18, 28, 30, 36, 56, 57, 101, 124, 141

Gila River Indian Community, 17

goat, 6, 47, 48, 50, 67, 211, 212

Goldwater, Michael, 151

gomphothere, 9, 12

gourds, 10, 36, 46

grapes, 48, 59, 64, 66, 72, 110, 115, 116, 122, 166, 205, 206, 218. See also wine

Green Chile Cheeseburger Trail, 225

Griffith, Jim, 51

grocery stores, 112, 178–80, 211, 220

Gulf of California, 39, 69, 73, 107, 217

Gulf of Mexico, 39, 217

Hadj Ali (Hi Jolly), 149, 150

hamburger, vii, 43, 73, 184, 185, 186, 187, 210, 217, 220. See also cheeseburger

Hand, George, 201–2

Harrison, Jim, 223

Harvey, Fred, 119–20, 177

Hatch, New Mexico, 38, 68, 69, 78, 144, 225

Haury, Emil, 8

Hayden, Julian, 3

High Rolls, New Mexico, 22–23, 39

Index

Hill, Jane, 28
Hines, Duncan, 183
Hohokam, vii, 8, 22, 25, 29, 30, 36, 55, 192
honey, xii, 38, 39, 43, 79, 121, 147, 193, 198,
    199
Hopi people, 16, 24, 27, 35, 36
horse, 2, 3, 8, 11, 13, 14, 48, 51, 57, 72, 93,
    138, 149
hot dog, vii, 185, 213, 214
huitlacoche (corn smut), 34–35, 212, 224
If He Hollers Let Him Go (novel by
    Chester Hines), 138

Indians and South Asians in Southwest,
    166, 168, 225
In-N-Out, 186
insects, 22, 28, 39, 76, 99, 216–17, 224
irrigation, 28, 36, 44, 55, 123–26, 162, 178
Italians in Southwest, 154–55, 156, 175,
    205–6, 211, 222

Jackson, Helen Hunt, 72
jaguar, 8, 11
Japanese in Southwest, 162–65, 168, 173,
    224
Jaquith, Waldo, 216
Jefferson, Thomas, 76, 88, 111, 197
Jews in Southwest, 143, 141–47, 151, 155,
    159, 189, 203

Kansas, x, xi, 92, 106, 132, 136
King, Thomas Starr, 115–16, 122
Kino, Eusebio Francisco, 55–57, 59, 63,
    64, 116
Kiowa-Tanoan people, 28, 36
Kokopelli, 29
kolache, 152, 153, 212
Korean cuisine, 170–72, 214
Kroc, Ray, 185–86

La Brea Tar Pits, California, 13
La Maravilla (novel by Alfredo Véa),
    77–79

Lankershim, Isaac, 143–44
Las Vegas, Nevada, xi, 107, 123, 160
Las Vegas, New Mexico, 120
Lebanese in Southwest, 147–50
lemon, 61, 116, 117, 133, 162, 175, 211
Leysath, Scott, 85
Los Angeles, California, 12, 13, 58, 60,
    77, 79, 101, 105, 106, 108, 115–17, 123,
    127, 130, 132, 139, 143, 146, 147, 152,
    154, 155, 158, 160, 163, 164, 167, 169–
    71, 172, 179, 181, 183, 186, 198, 203,
    205, 212, 214, 215, 221, 223, 225
Louisiana, x, 88, 90, 154, 157
Luby's, 120–21

Magoffin, Susan, 66–68
maize. *See* corn
mammoth, 1, 3, 8, 9, 11, 12, 13, 14
margarita, 194–95
mastodon, 9, 11, 13
Matson, Daniel, 28
McDonald's, 184–86
McJunkin, George, 8
mesquite, 19, 23, 31, 32, 39, 136, 206, 224
Mexicali, Baja California, Mexico, 160,
    161–62, 168, 224
migas, 71
migration, human, 1, 5–7, 10, 11, 13, 14,
    21, 28, 101, 130, 161, 166, 169, 171,
    203, 210
Mingus, Charles, 155
missions, Spanish, 56–59, 71–73, 113, 115,
    116–17, 121, 205
Mix, Thomas Hezekiah, 205–6
Montezuma, 24, 41, 44–46, 47, 54
Moor's Account, The (novel by Laila Lal-
    ami), 128–29
Morro Bay, California, 157, 223
mountain lion, 11
Murray Springs Clovis Site, Arizona, 14

nachos, 180–82
Native Seeds, 25, 36, 223

Navajo people, 7, 40, 68, 149, 170, 179, 225

Nevada, xi, 1, 107, 123, 160

New Mexico, x, xi, 2, 7, 8, 10, 14, 15, 16, 17, 20, 22, 27, 28, 29, 36, 55, 56, 70, 66, 67, 68, 70, 74, 78, 79, 90, 93, 94, 95, 96, 98, 102, 107, 113, 114, 115, 117, 120, 124, 129, 144, 147, 150, 158, 162, 170, 182, 186, 191, 192, 194, 201, 203, 210, 221, 222, 223, 225

New Mexico FoodShed Alliance, 223

nixtamalization, 27, 40

Nogales, Arizona, 141–43, 146, 155, 185

okra, 25, 130, 131

Old Salt Woman, 16–17

olive, 48, 61, 80, 121, 145, 175

Oñate, Juan de, 54, 68

onion, xii, 35, 55, 63, 64, 65, 66, 68, 69, 70, 71, 72, 77, 101, 147, 164, 182, 211, 214, 223

orange, 51, 59, 61, 63, 72, 116–18, 173, 194, 198

Orange Crush, 198–99

Oregon Trail, 98, 150

otter, 8, 11

oyster, 118–19, 120, 159, 213

panic grass, 25

peach, 55, 59, 61, 63, 64, 72, 102, 116

pear, 59, 64, 72, 110, 116

peas, 57, 63, 64, 130

pecan, 31, 32, 116, 144

Phoenix, Arizona, 16, 22, 36, 56, 75, 76, 100, 101, 123, 124, 168, 169, 190, 204, 206, 216, 223

Pico, Pio de Jesús, 127–28

Pie Town, New Mexico, 60, 225

pig, ix, 9, 48, 54, 71, 93, 121, 130, 135, 136, 159, 178, 192, 214, 217. See also pork

pineapple, 46, 147, 160, 225

pinyon nuts, 32–33

pistachio, 59

plum, 38, 55, 59, 63, 109, 110, 116

pork, xii, 66, 68, 69, 77, 78, 79, 80, 99, 121, 131, 133, 135, 136, 143, 147, 169, 172, 190, 211, 215, 225. See also pig

posole, 58, 68

potato, 37, 69, 75, 93, 99, 102, 109, 111–13, 120, 121, 130, 132, 146, 179, 182

prickly pear, 12, 31, 45, 55, 116, 195

pronghorn, 23, 31, 56, 58, 116

pulque, 46, 191, 193, 196

pumpkin, 43, 61, 64

purslane, 23, 76–77

Quartzsite, Arizona, 149–50

rabbit, 2, 21, 22, 38, 225

radish, ix, 47, 63, 211

railroad, 88, 92, 94, 102, 117, 118–19, 158, 166, 177, 213, 216

Rathje, William, 219

rice, viii, 26, 48, 49, 52, 61, 66, 67, 72, 79, 97, 98, 102, 126, 163, 165, 167, 170, 177, 180, 185, 215, 224

Rio Grande, 2, 14, 15, 16, 17, 23, 28, 39, 54, 55, 56, 68, 96, 113, 115, 117, 144, 204

rock art, 1, 29

Ronstadt, Frederick, 151

root beer, 184, 197, 198

Rubio, Ralph, 73–74

Sacramento Mountains, New Mexico, 22, 39

Sacramento Valley, California, 106

saguaro, 33–34, 191

Sahagún, Bernardino de, 38, 44

Sahara, 3–4, 6, 13, 50, 217

salsa, 45, 46, 47, 65, 78, 79, 114, 147, 148, 160, 179, 210, 211, 215

salt, 16, 17

Salt River, Arizona, 19, 36

San Antonio, New Mexico, 225

San Antonio, Texas, 31, 56, 65, 124, 132, 161, 181, 187, 198, 203, 204, 221

San Bernardino, California, 105, 107, 117, 185, 186
San Francisco, California, 56, 118, 154, 157, 158, 159, 168, 205, 223
San Gabriel, California, 71, 72, 115–17, 127
Sanchez, Guadalupe, 12
Santa Barbara, California, x, 115, 157, 205
Santa Fe, New Mexico, 23, 55, 66, 75, 79, 94, 98, 118, 119, 120, 129, 182, 204, 225
Santo Domingo Pueblo, 16
scallops, 213
Sea of Cortez. *See* Gulf of California
Sea of Grass (novel by Conrad Richter), 96–97
Sears, Richard Warren, 177–78
Serra, Junípero, 57, 116, 205
sheep, 6, 11, 22, 48, 54, 56, 72, 122, 146, 149
shrimp, 69, 79, 213, 218
slavery, 31, 48, 56, 57, 87–88, 90–92, 128, 129, 130, 131, 135
smilodon, 8, 11, 13, 14
soft drinks, 197–99
son-of-a-bitch stew, 70
Sonora, Mexico, 12, 17, 21, 25, 31, 48, 56, 69, 74, 75, 77, 116, 141, 151, 162, 194, 204, 210, 213
Sonoran Desert, 7, 8, 19, 33, 34, 37, 191, 218
Sonoran hot dog, 213–14
Southern cuisine, 130–34, 179
Southwest, defined geographically, ix–xii
Spanish in Southwest, viii, ix, 17, 21, 24, 31–32, 37, 38, 41, 43, 44, 45, 47, 48, 50–51, 56–61, 65, 66, 72, 83, 84, 90, 91–93, 94, 102, 103, 105, 113–15, 117, 121, 127, 147, 194, 204, 205, 218
squash, 35, 36, 38, 39, 46, 47, 55, 61, 74
Stumberg, Louis, 187

sugar, 31, 37, 48, 45, 63, 67, 79, 90, 98, 99, 109, 116, 130, 143, 153, 156, 191, 192, 193, 225
sushi, 163–65, 167, 215, 224

Taco Bell, 186–87
taco, vii–viii, ix, xii, 44–46, 64, 69, 73, 79, 114, 147–48, 165, 170, 171, 184, 186–87, 210, 211, 213–14, 216, 225
tacos al pastor, 147–48
tamale, vii, 24, 25, 38, 39, 44, 45, 52, 75, 79–80, 132, 133, 151, 154, 187, 190, 210, 211, 225
tepary beans, 35, 215, 224
tequila, 68, 192, 193, 193, 196, 199, 200
Tewa Pueblo, 23
Texas, x, xi, 2, 7, 11, 12, 14, 15, 21, 23, 28, 31–33, 36, 48, 49, 50, 54, 65, 69, 70, 71, 77, 79, 80, 83, 90, 91, 92, 93, 96, 99, 100, 101, 107, 113, 114, 115, 117, 121, 124, 129, 130, 133, 134, 135, 136, 137, 143, 144, 145, 146, 150, 151, 152, 153, 154, 157, 158, 161, 166, 169, 180, 181, 182, 186, 187, 191, 194, 198, 202, 203, 204, 210, 211, 212, 215, 224
Thai cuisine, 170
tiswin, 191, 199–200, 202, 225
tlacoyo, 34, 35, 44–46, 187
tobacco, 23, 27, 46, 48, 54, 91, 92, 111, 121
Tohono O'odham, vii, 17, 29, 33–34, 56, 59, 93, 215
tomato, ix, xii, 37, 38, 44, 46, 64, 66, 67, 111, 113, 114, 120, 122, 136, 163, 166, 211, 214, 216
tortilla, xii, 35, 38, 64, 66, 71, 74, 75, 77, 79, 102, 103, 147, 148, 154, 179, 180, 182, 190, 210, 211, 225
Trader Joe's, 180, 222
True Grit (novel by Charles Portis), 80
Tucson, Arizona, viii, 52, 64, 75, 77, 79, 92, 103, 107, 130, 134, 142, 146, 151, 154, 158, 161, 163, 169, 171, 184, 186,

189, 192, 201, 203, 206, 211, 212, 214, 218, 219, 221
Tumacacori Mission, 59
turkey, 23, 38, 40, 44, 50, 70, 143
Twain, Mark, 99, 118

University of Arizona, 114, 219
Urrea, Luis Alberto, xii
Utah, x, xi, 28, 40, 98, 120, 162, 187
Uto-Aztecan languages, 7, 16, 23, 28, 29

Vallejo, Guadalupe, 72–73
vanilla, 46, 67
venison, 38, 85, 132, 134
Ventana Cave, Arizona, 8
Vietnamese in Southwest, 169–70, 215

walnut, 59, 63, 127, 141
waste, food, 219–21

watermelon, 34, 59, 61, 63
wheat, viii, ix, 24, 43, 47, 48, 51, 55, 56, 57, 61, 63, 64, 66, 72, 73, 75, 121, 125, 127, 143, 144, 210
Wheat, Margaret, 33
Whole Foods, 180, 222
wine, 49, 51, 66, 85, 115, 152, 196, 204–6
wolf, dire, 8
World War II, 122, 129, 138–39, 161, 163, 165, 180, 187, 188, 189, 190

Yaqui people, 75
Yokohama, California (memoir by Toshio Mori), 162–63
Yuma, Arizona, 107, 122

Zepeda, Ofelia, 34
Zwinger, Ann, 126